60 SIMPLE TIPS TO STAY HEALTHY AND FIT

Weight Loss, Exercise and Healthy Eating

Lewis Demilade Babatope

CONTENTS

INTRODUCTION

"60 Simple Tips to Stay Healthy and Fit" provides the knowledge you need to achieve and maintain a healthy lifestyle. Can you relate to the daily struggle of trying to eat healthy and stay fit?, if so, this book is for you. It gives you the knowledge you need to maintain good health and prevent diseases.

It is a simple fact that, if you are to lose weight, you need to use up more calories than you take in. Maintaining a proper diet can seem like a challenging task, yet it is an important part of a healthy living plan. Eating nutrient-dense foods in their natural state is a key factor in maintaining optimal wellness. Do you ever drive past the gym and wonder if working out is really worth the effort? Exercise offers truly life-changing results if you're willing to put in the effort required.

Are you ready for your transformation? Do not let life pass you by, learn to control it and live it like you are meant to! Remember, this is the only body you have.

ABOUT THE AUTHOR

Lewis Demilade Babatope, the author of **"60 Simple Tips to Stay Healthy and Fit"** founded the website "www.myhealthfuldiet.com." He is a firm believer in helping people quit their inactive and unhealthy lifestyle.

He promotes concepts of health and wellness to people struggling to make a permanent lifestyle change. He also offers readers with strategies and tips needed to turn their lives around by maintaining a healthy diet and exercise routine - two important things needed to live a long and prosperous life. His aim is to provide the resources needed to prevent diseases.

His book and website are his ways of helping people fight the urge to live an unhealthy lifestyle. He has compiled his years of knowledge on various health and fitness topics in his book and website to provide the ultimate resources needed to bring a much awaited transformation.

DISCLAIMER

The information contained in this book is for educational purpose only. The purpose of this book is to promote the understanding of various diet and fitness topics. It is not intended to be a substitute for professional medical advice, diagnosis or treatment.

Always seek the advice of your physician or other qualified health care provider with any questions you may have regarding a medical condition or treatment before undertaking a new health regimen, and never disregard professional medical advice or delay seeking it because of what you read in this book.

PART A: WEIGHT LOSS TIPS

It's a simple fact that, if you are to lose weight, you need to use up more calories than you take in. This section will provide you with effective weight loss tips that you'll need to stay fit.

TIP #1: LOSE WEIGHT WITHOUT DIETING BY MAKING SEVEN LIFESTYLE CHANGES

Dieting conjures up images of deprivation. You sacrifice your taste buds and the foods you like to lose weight. And how long do you stay on this diet? Will you ever eat a chocolate bar again? To compound matters, despite all the pain, you are likely to regain the weight you lose.

According to a study published in American Psychologist in 2007, about 80 percent of people on a diet plan regain their lost weight - and even gain more - over five years. Wouldn't it be better to find a way to lose weight, and keep it off, without dieting? And there is. The following tips will aid in your weight loss.

1.   Watch the amount you eat
You don't need to avoid your favorite foods, but watch how much you eat. Use a small plate and serve small portions. When going to a party, eat a healthy snack beforehand to avoid heaping your plate. Wait for about 20 minutes before refilling your plate after a serving, and drink some water. According to nutritionists, your brain takes about 20 minutes to register fullness.

2.   Eat a protein at every meal
Make a lean or low-fat protein a component of every meal and snack. Refreshments containing nuts, peanut butter, low-fat yogurt, and lean meats keep you feeling full for longer so you're unlikely to overeat at your next meal. Snacking also keeps your blood sugar levels stable to avoid gorging at your next meal.

3. Eat slowly and concentrate on your food

Savor every bite. Take your time with every mouthful. Don't read, watch TV, or work while eating. Concentrate on eating. Enjoy your food. Research findings published in the British Journal of Nutrition suggest that being distracted can make you ignore signs of being full.

4. Load up on fruits and vegetables

Eat lots of low-calorie, high fiber fruits and vegetables to replace high fat, high sugar, and high-calorie foods. Consider starting lunch or dinner with a bowl of soup or a vegetable salad. This will drive away the pangs of hunger, making you eat less than you would otherwise.

5. Get moving

Walk, walk, and walk. Speed walk, walk to the store, park your car and walk to work. Pace while you talk on the phone, run up and down the stairs. Just get moving. Combine cardio and resistant training to burn off the calories and tone up your body. If you are so inclined, get a pedometer to record the number of steps you take per day. Try to increase the steps by the day.

6. Choose your drinks wisely

Quench your thirst with plain water. Skip sugary, flavored drinks that offer nothing but calories and can lead to weight gain. These drinks also raise the risk of type 2 diabetes. Take no more than a small glass of 100% fruit juice per day. Coffee and tea are fine, but go easy on the sugar and cream. Drink a glass or two a day maximum of low fat or skim milk, as it is high in calories.

7. Get enough sleep

Sleep restores the body - both mentally and physically. Your body needs sleep for all-round health. A study by neurologist Thorsten Kahnt, published in October 2019 in eLife, a scientific journal, indicated that when you are sleep-deprived you snack more, and on unhealthy foods. When you're sleep-deprived, you crave sugary and fat-laden foods.

Bottom line

When you make these adjustments in your life, they soon become second nature and you'll not even remember you made them to lose weight. The weight that you lose will stay off, as opposed to going on a diet that you will throw out of the window within no time.

TIP #2: FIVE MEDICAL BENEFITS OF LOSING WEIGHT

Doctors around the world advise overweight patients to lose weight. Even when people feel fine, carrying excess weight can have harmful effects on the body. Approaching or achieving an ideal weight can reverse or lessen these effects and even prevent some health conditions. Here are some of the medical benefits associated with losing weight.

Lower blood pressure
Losing 5 percent to 10 percent of your body weight can lower your blood pressure by five points -- a significant step for people with moderate hypertension. Reducing your sodium intake and eating a healthy diet can lower your blood pressure even more. Ask your doctor about low-calorie and heart-healthy diet plans.

Lower risk of diabetes
Losing weight can benefit your blood sugar level. When you are overweight, your body becomes less sensitive to insulin, a condition known as insulin resistance. Insulin resistance is a major predictor of diabetes. A 7-percent decrease in your weight coupled with some physical activity, such as walking, can reduce your risk of developing type 2 diabetes.

Reduced sleep apnea
Sleep apnea is a condition which causes sufferers to wake up multiple times during the night to gasp for air. Interrupting normal sleep cycles can lead to high blood pressure, memory problems, and exhaustion. Being overweight can make sleep apnea worse. Losing weight can significantly reduce the frequency of sleep apnea episodes and improve overall health.

Fewer heart issues

Overweight bodies require more heart capacity to pump a greater volume of blood. This extra work enlarges the heart cavity and makes the heart muscles thicker. It can also lead to heart failure. Reducing your weight by 10 percent can lower your risk of developing a heart condition, regardless of whether you lose weight quickly or if you lose it slowly but consistently.

Lower cholesterol

Losing weight can increase your good cholesterol and lower your bad cholesterol. It only takes a modest 5- to 10-percent weight loss to raise your good cholesterol (HDL) by five points. A high level of HDL indicates a lower risk of developing heart issues.

These are just a few of the medical benefits associated with weight loss, but they are some of the most important. When you can't get motivated to exercise or stick to a diet plan, just remember how even a small weight loss can benefit your health.

TIP #3: TEN WEIGHT-LOSS TIPS TO CONSIDER AS YOU AGE

Some people can maintain a healthy body weight in their youth and through the early years of adulthood with ease. Other people have struggled with the number on the scale for as long as they can remember. Eventually, however, there comes a time in nearly everyone's life where age and the aging process start to wreak havoc with muscle tone, fat distribution, and overall body weight. Whether hormones, lifestyle choices or just overall laziness is causing the problem, there is a noticeable change that many people want to avoid if at all possible.

While you can't stop the clock or turn back the ravages of time, there are some changes you can, and should, make to help maintain or regain that sleek look of youth.

1. First of all, you have to acknowledge reality. You aren't a teenager anymore. You may not even be able to lay claim to young adulthood. If you've passed the age of 40, you are flirting with middle age. Accepting this fact, however, doesn't mean you have to give in to what seems inevitable; it just means you have to face a new set of challenges. Don't worry. There are plenty of ways to fight back.

2. Fruits and vegetables were always an important part of your healthy diet, but they should take on a whole new meaning as your age creeps up. Fruits and vegetables will always give you more bang for your calorie intake than just about any other food or food group. They provide sufficient nutrients with minimal calories, and they can be quite filling as well, allowing you to feel satiated sooner.

3.   Breakfast is more important than ever if you are trying to control your weight and your food intake. Whole grain cereals, along with protein from eggs or yogurt will provide a full stomach a lot longer than a cheese Danish or pancakes with a side of hash browns.

4.   Some people swear by the philosophy of eating a heftier meal at lunch time and then cutting back on their food consumption at dinner. The idea is to have more hours to burn off some of those mid-day calories. When you consume your calories, however, is not as critical as how many you take in throughout the day. The choice is still yours. Regardless of how you structure your meals, it's always a good idea to stop eating when you've finished dinner. Midnight snacks can be detrimental to your waistline.

5.   If you haven't been doing so up until this point in your life, start preparing and eating more of your meals at home. Restaurant meals are a minefield of hidden fat, sodium, sugar and calories. The best way to monitor your food intake is by preparing most of your meals yourself, with ingredients you recognize and portions you control.

6.   Of course, you know the importance of portion control. Nutritionists have been preaching it for years. There are two things to understand about the concept: 1) a normal portion is probably less than what you have been accustomed to eating most of your life; 2) you should eat that smaller portion and never return for seconds. That second helping will defeat the purpose of minding your amounts.

7.   Learn to eat without multi-tasking. Savor your food. Appreciate what you are doing for your body. Distractions such as your cell phone, the television or your computer make it easy to eat more while enjoying it less. Share your meals with a loved one or

friend whenever possible to make the dining experience rewarding and healthy.

8.   Treat water as the elixir of life that it is. Make water your drink of choice as much as possible. Sodas and alcoholic beverages should be treats, much like chocolate cake for dessert. It's a scary statistic that many people consume a quarter or more of their daily calories from what they drink instead of what they eat.

9.   You may think you're too busy to work out, and you may be right. If that's the case for you, consider the eventual outcome. Exercise burns calories. Exercise tones your body. Exercise clears your mind. Exercise keeps vital organs operating at peak efficiency. Lack of exercise reduces all of these outcomes for you as you age. Now, are you still sure you are too busy to exercise?

10. Getting a good night's sleep is about more than not being tired each day. Sleep, much like exercise, rejuvenates the body. Poor sleep is associated with weight gain, as well. If stress, medications or physical problems interfere with getting adequate rest, you owe it to yourself to address these issues with a doctor.

Weight gain is not an inevitable consequence of aging. You have to learn to adjust your life and your habits to make the most of every aspect of your life. You have many more decades of life to live. You should do so while feeling and looking your best. Weight management will help you achieve both goals.

TIP #4: LOSE WEIGHT WITH
APPLE CIDER VINEGAR

Apple cider vinegar is an incredibly powerful natural aid to weight loss, and has been applauded by people all over the world for its healing and nurturing properties. Its acidic nature can also help keep skin balanced, improve liver functions and encourage the growth of good gut bacteria.

One of the better-known uses for apple cider vinegar is to aid weight loss by managing and controlling the appetite. Its sweet yet acidic taste lends itself perfectly for use in low-fat home-made salad dressings and stir fries, and small amounts can be included in most sauces without altering their taste.

The most powerful and beneficial way to introduce your body to apple cider vinegar and kick start its weight-loss abilities is to use this tried-and-tested recipe for a morning drink:

- Pour an 8 ounce glass of warm water. Make sure the water is filtered and as pure as possible, and the temperature not hot, but warmer than room temperature.

- Add one tablespoon of organic apple cider vinegar and stir.

- Add lemon juice, honey or tea to taste.

Drink the mixture as soon as possible after waking in the morning, on an empty stomach. Allow at least half an hour for the vinegar to make it through your system before having a meal. Many people experience a dramatic loss in appetite on the first day; however, give it a week or so if you are not seeing immediate effects.

Most people dislike the thought of drinking diluted vinegar. However, good brands will taste more sweet than bitter, like salt and vinegar chips. You can alter the amount of vinegar used if you prefer it stronger or weaker, but be aware that too-high acidity in the diet can lead to stomachache and other complications. If you prefer it normal strength or weaker, you can enjoy the drink up to twice a day if you like with no ill effects.

You will see a reduction in appetite, but also might notice other changes in your body. Your digestion may improve, your skin get clearer, and your sweet tooth may be lessened. These results will ensure your diet remains balanced and moderate, and will also aid healthy weight loss when combined with regular daily exercise.

TIP #5: COULD THE WAY YOUR BODY PROCESSES FOOD BE WHY YOU ARE STRUGGLING TO LOSE WEIGHT?

It's a simple fact that, if you are to lose weight, you need to use up more calories than you take in. That is why doctors and nutrition experts identify good and bad foods for weight loss, where good foods tend to be lower-calorie foods. Anybody who has been on a diet will be familiar with the foods that are considered bad for weight loss. These are foods that contain high levels of fat, starch or sugar. The problem for many people is that they struggle to lose weight even when they stick to the supposedly good foods.

What is happening?
It turns out that how the body processes food is more complex than was previously thought. There is widespread agreement that food is converted to sugar that is carried around in the blood to provide energy for bodily functions. Any unused sugar is converted to fat and stored. The prevailing thought is that cutting out the so-called bad foods, which are high in calories, must reduce the amount of fat stored.

Some scientists are now beginning to call that conclusion into question, or at least suggest that it does not always apply. It has emerged that eating some types of fatty food does not increase calorie intake as much as was once thought, because some types of fat, such as those in unprocessed meat products, are difficult to break down. Although these meat products may be high in calories, a significant portion of their calories are excreted rather than converted to stored fat.

One of the most surprising discoveries comes from research carried out by the Weitzmann Institute in Israel, which showed remarkably different responses in people who had the same food intake. Volunteers had their blood sugar levels monitored every few minutes over the course of a week. The expectation would have been that blood sugar levels would rise higher after consumption of sugary foods than after consumption of so-called healthier foods. Researchers were surprised to find that the expected increase in blood sugar levels did not always occur. Some of the most surprising episodes were where eating tomatoes caused a bigger rise in blood sugar levels than eating ice cream, or eating bananas caused higher levels than eating cookies.

Spikes in blood sugar levels, no matter how they are caused, will lead to fat storage if the calories are not used up. The unavoidable conclusion is that sticking to healthy foods may not guarantee weight loss for every person.

Does the research mean you should abandon your diet?
Definitely not! The basic premise that you must burn more calories than you consume in order to lose weight remains true. It would be foolish in the extreme to conclude from the Weitzmann research that eating loads of ice cream or cookies will help you lose weight. What you can conclude from the research is that you may need to experiment with your diet to figure out which foods suit you best in terms of losing weight.

You could also experiment with the times you eat, such as having your main meal earlier in the day. Similarly, try exercising at different times. Going for a brisk walk after a meal can burn up blood sugar, whereas being sedentary after eating can cause fat storage.

The mantra that you should stick to a balanced, nutritious diet still holds. By definition, a balanced diet is one that does not contain too much of the same type of food. With a balanced diet, you will not be eating too much of any foods that you have an unusual response to in terms of your blood sugar levels. It is also advisable to avoid processed foods as much as possible. When foods are processed, their chemical structure is often changed, making them easier to digest. That means the body can extract more sugar from processed food than from natural ones.

The Bottom line
Everybody can lose weight, but diets that work for other people may not work for you. If your dieting efforts have not yielded the expected results, try to change some of the healthy things that you have been eating, and look for other lifestyle changes that could influence the way your body handles food.

TIP #6: FIVE PROVEN WEIGHT-LOSS FOODS YOU SHOULD BE EATING

Losing weight can be a long process, but if you incorporate these foods into your diet, you may see results faster than you expected. In addition to exercise and healthy lifestyle choices like getting enough rest, drinking enough water, and having a positive outlook on life, these five foods can accelerate your progress in a healthy and tasty way.

1. Matcha

Unlike standard green tea, matcha is the entirety of the green tea leaf ground into a powder. This allows you to ingest the complete plant, which provides more benefit than the leaves steeped in hot water. One study conducted by the American Journal of Clinical Nutrition showed that drinking green tea increases the body's calorie-burning efficiency by about 400 percent; it burns more body fat overall than other sources of fuel and increases your endurance during a workout. Therefore, if you're looking for more efficient workout sessions, matcha is the perfect food to eat just before a routine.

Matcha's high concentration of antioxidants far outweigh that of pomegranates, goji berries, or blueberries, and it has the antioxidant power of 10 cups of regular green tea. The great thing about matcha is that it can be added to just about anything. Try it in a smoothie or with warm coconut, almond, or rice milk.

2. Avocado

In times past, fat was considered evil. In the case of avocados, however, fats can be a great tool for weight loss. Avocados contain oleic acid, a monosaturated fat that is usually burned before carbohydrates. This can lead to a leaner body over time. Avocados also help your body absorb nutrients from other foods you eat along with it, and because your body has acquired more nutrients from your meal, you stay fuller longer. Avocados can serve as a complement to many meals because of their mild, buttery taste and texture. Try having a few slices on your sandwiches, add them to omelets, or garnish your chili and soups with them.

3. Oatmeal

Oatmeal may sound unexciting, but don't knock this American breakfast staple. It's full of fiber, which helps to curb hunger by keeping you satiated longer. A newer phenomenon, overnight oatmeal, is a handy way to incorporate these whole grains into your diet plan. This method involves mixing a serving of oats with other ingredients and storing them in the fridge until morning. Starting your day off with this heart-healthy food is a great way to kick-start your weight loss.

4. Eggs

Eggs were once considered unhealthy because of their effect on cholesterol, but recent studies have shed some light on this old myth. Once thought to increase cholesterol levels, many recent studies have proven that eggs decrease your LDL cholesterol (the bad kind) and increase your HDL (the good kind). Full of vitamins and nutrients essential to your body, eggs are primarily composed of fat and protein, two macros that aid in keeping you full for longer.

5. Quinoa

Quinoa is another source of healthy protein that will curb hunger. The ancient Incans referred to it as the "mother of all grains," a sentiment now shared by modern societies around the world. It is more fiber-dense than all other grains, which means a serving of it will work hand in hand with its protein content to reduce hunger. Try quinoa in a stir fry, or in soups or casseroles. They add a satisfying crunch to meals, and can even be used as a breading.

You have to make a lot of choices when you're trying to lose weight, and picking the correct foods is essential to your success. You can't go wrong including any of the above-mentioned foods in a balanced meal plan. With these foods in your arsenal, you can break away from conventional advice and start taking your health into your own hands.

TIP #7: FOUR DANGEROUS WEIGHT-LOSS METHODS YOU MUST AVOID

As much as you would like to lose weight quickly, some weight loss strategies do more harm than good. Extreme measures aren't necessarily the most effective, and some can even put your health at risk. Regardless of your weight loss goals, losing weight should improve your health, not make it worse. Here are 4 weight loss strategies that can harm your health

1. Weight Loss Drugs
Many drugs, both prescription and over-the-counter, claim to help people lose weight. While some are more effective than others, many so-called weight loss drugs contain dangerous chemicals that can threaten your health. "Metabolism boosters" and "fat burners" are questionable at best and are not regulated by the Food and Drug Administration. Stimulants, water pills and appetite suppressants have little effect on body fat and can have many harmful effects, especially on overweight people. Even the prescription weight loss pill Fen-phen was pulled from the market after it caused fatal hypertension and heart valve problems. Before resorting to drugs - which you should only do with a doctor's supervision - give natural methods a serious effort and spare yourself the health complications.

2. Over-Exercising
Over-exercising can have serious side effects, particularly in people who are in poor physical condition. While burning calories is important, over-exercising can do more harm than good. When muscles- including the heart- work hard, they develop microscopic tears that require rest periods to heal. Without adequate rest periods, the heart can develop scarring called

cardiac fibrosis and can also enlarge, creating a greater risk for a heart attack during exercise. Too much intense or prolonged exercise can also make your body produce too much cortisol as a response to stress. Excess cortisol can weaken your immune system, interfere with sleep and cause chronic inflammation throughout your body.

Additionally, working beyond your capacity increases your risk for injury. Pain and even extremely sore muscles can prevent you from working out at all for days or weeks, so it can be counterproductive. The intense exercise you see on television weight loss shows is staged for dramatic effect and isn't healthy. It's more important to exercise correctly and consistently than to overdo it every day.

3. Skipping Meals

While you can gain weight by overeating, regularly skipping meals is not always a good way to lose weight. Skipping too many meals can sometimes make you even hungrier and more likely to overeat when you finally do. Going too long between meals can also affect your blood sugar, particularly if you are diabetic, and can cause problems if you have low blood pressure. It can also make you feel sluggish and less motivated to exercise or do anything that requires physical effort. Skipping meals until you're extremely hungry and then overeating just encourages an unhealthy relationship with food that ultimately, won't help you lose weight any faster.

It's easier, safer and more effective to develop good eating habits, such as limiting portion sizes, eating on a regular schedule, avoiding high-calorie, low-nutrient snacks and ensuring that your diet is balanced and complete.

4. Smoking

Some people smoke to suppress hunger or as a substitute for snacking. Others are afraid to quit, believing that they will gain weight if they do. When people gain weight after they quit smoking, it's because they changed their eating habits. Smoking has no direct effect on weight loss, and is also dangerous to your health. It raises your blood pressure, increases your heart rate, constricts your blood vessels, raises your cholesterol and increases your chances of a heart attack or stroke. It has many of the same dangerous effects as excess weight, so it's not worth it to smoke for the sake of weight loss. If you need help controlling your appetite, use natural methods such as eating more fiber, avoiding insulin spikes, drinking more water and exercising regularly.

Permanent weight loss is a process, and it takes time to get results. With so many safe weight loss methods, you don't need to use one that's harmful to your health, even if it works quickly. If you are losing weight for health reasons, such as to lower your blood pressure, control diabetes or to help with chronic pain, don't use a method that will compound existing health problems. Traditional methods such as calorie counting, eating sensibly and increasing exercise have worked for millions of people and they can work for you.

TIP #8: WEIGHT LOSS SUCCESS WITH YOGURT

Losing Weight comes surprisingly easy for many people, and exceedingly hard for others. How is it possible that two people who have similar physical builds, eat the same number of calories, and do the same amount of exercise have such different weight loss outcomes? The secret may lie in what foods are being consumed. For example, if one person consumes yogurt daily, and the other person does not, the person who does include yogurt in their diet will likely lose more weight faster than the one who does not. Can yogurt really help you to lose weight?

We hear a lot about probiotics and their health benefits. A probiotic is a good bacterium. Antibiotics are used to combat harmful bacteria, but can also kill off the beneficial bacteria in the process. You may have seen probiotic supplements in the vitamin aisle at your local pharmacy. You probably also noticed the high price tag for those probiotics. Luckily, you can regenerate the good bacteria your body needs by consuming yogurt. If you eat yogurt every day, you should have no need of probiotic supplements.

One way that yogurt helps you to lose weight is by helping with the digestion process. This is done with the common inclusion of three different probiotic bacterium: Bulgaricus, Streptococcus Thermophilus, and Lactobacillus. There are usually other probiotics added as well, which makes the yogurt more beneficial. This good bacterium helps to break food down in a more efficient manner and also improves the way that your body absorbs nutrients from the foods you consume as they are being digested.

Yogurt is made from milk, which contains protein. This gives your body some of the protein that is needed to lose weight even if you do not eat a lot of meat. Additionally, most people who are lactose intolerant tolerate yogurt very well, and yogurt actually helps to combat lactose intolerance.

Yogurt can be bought in bulk, but the smaller one-serving containers are recommended because of their convenience. These small containers make awesome, quick snacks or healthy desserts. If you do not have time for a full lunch, eat one or two containers of yogurt instead.

If you want to add beneficial yogurt to your daily diet, make sure that you are buying the correct type of yogurt. The brand is not important. However, live active cultures are important if you want to benefit from yogurt. The label should specifically say that the product has live active cultures. Do not be fooled by a product that states it contains at least 100 million live active cultures. This is the minimum required by the National Yogurt Association.

When you stand in front of the yogurt section in your grocery store, resist the urge to flee as you are confronted by all the different types, flavors, and brands of yogurt that are available. It can be quite overwhelming. You should avoid frozen yogurt, as it does not have as many live cultures as non-frozen yogurt. Greek yogurt will have more protein, but less calcium. It is also higher in calories than other types.

Keep to traditional types of yogurt and choose one that is "light" or lower in calories and sugars. If you are vegetarian or vegan, you cannot go wrong with a soy yogurt. Additionally, yogurt will help you to feel full faster if it contains small bits of fruit in it. Start with your favorite plain yogurt, and then experiment with different nuts and fruits at home to make and keep it interesting.

Yogurt is a very healthy choice to add to your weight loss plan, and it really can help you to lose weight. However, you should use caution. Most people enjoy the taste of yogurt, and like anything else, if you eat too much of it, you can affect your weight loss efforts.

TIP #9: HOW TO EAT MORE FIBER
AND DROP THE POUNDS

The basics of successful weight loss will always boil down to reducing the number of calories you consume while increasing the amount of exercise you take. However, eating less is only half the story when it comes to battling the calories. A healthy diet can go a long way toward making your body process your food a lot more efficiently, turning it into healthy energy rather than storing it up as extra pounds.

Fiber is one powerful part of a healthy diet for better weight loss. Dietary fiber helps to control the digestion process, smoothing out the peaks and troughs in blood sugar levels which can lead to those irresistible hunger pangs. It is also more difficult to digest than highly processed foods, so you feel fuller for longer, and indeed much of the fiber you eat passes straight through your system without adding to your calorie intake at all.

Given these powerful weight loss benefits, how can you easily increase the amount of fiber you consume in your daily diet?

Make a Habit of Wholemeal
Wholemeal grains contain far more fiber than processed white grains, so try and substitute them whenever you can. This means opting for wholemeal or wholegrain bread rather than plain white, choosing brown or wild rice instead of the more common polished varieties, and even buying wholemeal pasta for those quick, healthy, mid-week suppers.

Go Green and Leafy

Dark, leafy vegetables such as kale, spinach, and broccoli are all rich in fiber, as well as being packed with vitamins and antioxidants which are highly beneficial for overall health. Although you may be used to eating your greens as a side dish, they can become the star of the show in stir-fries, soups, and hearty warm salads.

Lovely Legumes

Beans, peas, and lentils are all highly nutritious, high in fiber, and also an excellent source of protein for those wishing to cut down on meat. They're equally delicious in warming winter casseroles or super summer salads.

Beautiful Berries

Berries of all kinds, from raspberries to redcurrants, are excellent sources of dietary fiber. They're also high in vitamin C, and their sweetness provides a welcome change when you've sworn off other, less healthy dessert options.

Nutritious Nuts

Nuts and seeds make a healthy snack for when hunger pangs strike, but they're also full of vital fiber. Eat them as they are, add a small handful chopped to salads for an oriental twist, or sprinkle over your breakfast cereal for a sustaining start to the day.

Bring on the Bran

Lastly, bran has long been a popular source of quick and tasty dietary fiber. Whether baked into your favorite low-fat muffin recipe or eaten as a healthy breakfast cereal, bran is one of the best fiber providers you'll find.

No matter which diet plan you're following, increasing your fiber intake will boost your efforts toward weight loss success -

and bring you many other health benefits alongside.

TIP #10: HOW TO CHOOSE MEAL REPLACEMENT SHAKES FOR EFFECTIVE WEIGHT LOSS RESULTS

Beyond the many diet plan fashions which come and go, there's one underlying truth to weight loss. To shed the pounds, you need to eat fewer calories while taking more exercise.

The problem with cutting back on calorie intake is that you can feel constantly hungry and unsatisfied, making any diet plan an uphill struggle when tempting treats are never far away. One great solution to this problem is a meal replacement shake, which provides the nutrition you need in a physically filling format without the excess calories which will sabotage your diet.

But what should you look for when choosing between the many different shakes on the market? Here are the three main areas to consider.

1) Basic Shake Types for Different Diets
Depending on the type of diet plan you're following, you might need a different type of shake to best fit in. There are five basic kinds to choose from.

- Plant-based shakes are mostly or entirely made from vegetable proteins, and are ideal for those following a vegetarian or vegan diet. However, check on the ingredients list before buying if you have any food allergies, as these shakes often contain traces of nuts, soy, hemp, or other sources which some people find difficult to digest.

- Keto-friendly shakes are low in carbs to suit those following keto-based diet plans.

- Paleo-friendly shakes place the emphasis on wholefood ingredients with as little extra processing as possible.

- Low-sugar shakes don't rely on sweetness to be palatable, and so are particularly low in calories as well as suitable for those with blood sugar issues.

- Very low-calorie shakes are great for reducing your daily calorie intake, but can leave you feeling hungry and lacking in energy. It's usually best to try these once you've got into the meal replacement routine, rather than making them your first choice when starting out.

2) Protein Sources

Most shakes rely on concentrated proteins to leave you feeling satisfied, and these proteins come from a few typical sources.
- Whey protein is the most common, and is made from milk. It's easy to digest and can assist in turning fat into lean, toned muscle, but isn't suitable for vegans or people with lactose intolerance.

- Casein is another protein that's derived from milk, but it's digested and metabolized much more slowly than whey protein. This makes it a good choice if working out is a large part of your weight loss routine, as it helps muscle recovery over a longer period.

- Soy protein is made from soybeans and is great for vegans and vegetarians. It provides complex proteins containing the full range of amino acids for all-round nutritional health, but has a couple of drawbacks. Many soy shakes are made from genetically modified ingredients, so choose an organic product if you want to avoid this. Also, excessive soy can have an estrogen-like effect on the body, so all soy-based products should be used with care.

- Pea protein is another complex source that's suitable for vegans. What's more, its high fiber levels can produce stronger feelings of fullness, to keep hunger at bay for longer.

- Brown rice protein is a good dairy-free source, but doesn't offer the full-spectrum of amino acids. If you use only brown rice shakes, then make sure the rest of your diet contains a full nutritional range to make up for this lack.

- Hemp protein is extremely rich in omega-3 fatty acids, which promote joint, brain, and cardiovascular health. However, it's not a good source of most other amino acids, so should be used as part of a fully balanced diet.

3) Added Extras

While in most cases unprocessed wholefoods are the most desirable for health, when it comes to meal replacement shakes sometimes a few added extras can be beneficial.

- Added fiber increases feelings of fullness while also promoting better digestive health.

- Added vitamins and minerals can help make up for any nutritional deficiencies a restricted diet can cause.

- Added superfood blends can bring the particular benefits of mushrooms, kale, spinach, and other ingredients, without the natural tastes and textures that are off-putting to some people.

- Added probiotics can help promote all-round digestive health, as well as providing support to the immune system.

While all these options can make choosing your meal replacement shake a little tricky, it also means there's plenty to try if your first choices don't work out as you'd hoped. By refining the exact type of shake your body needs, you can home in on a meal replacement routine that works for both your diet plan and your overall health.

PART B: EXERCISE TIPS

You need to put a spring into your step to become more alive, energetic, and confident. Exercise will definitely do that for you. This section will help you establish fitness goals, teach you different exercises, and make exercise something you love instead of hate.

TIP #11: THE AMAZING PHYSICAL AND MENTAL BENEFITS OF WALKING

Walking sounds like a boring exercise, just putting one foot in front of the other. As the saying goes, though, "big things come in small packages." Walking is one of the calmest and yet most beneficial forms of exercise. While not everyone is able to "walk," the same goes for those who use wheelchairs. As long as you're doing the repeated movement for locomotion, you'll see the benefits of walking. Beyond its physical pros, walking can also be incredible for mental health. Here are some of these benefits in more detail.

General Wellbeing

As a general rule of thumb, any kind of exercise can promote general wellbeing. However, like swimming, walking is one of the most gentle and accessible forms of exercise. It depends on your ability, but as long as you're moving mechanically and have an accessible path, it shouldn't matter whether you're walking on your feet or using a wheelchair with your arms.

Walking is very gentle and can be coupled with calming scenery. When you walk for a good amount of time, you're doing exercise that may not even feel like exercise. For example, if you enjoy hiking and live near a beautiful forest, walking can be an incredible form of exercise. You're improving your physical state by continuously moving, which releases endorphins like when you run, and you're definitely improving your mental state by surrounding yourself with beautiful, natural scenery. Overall, as long as you choose a path and destination that makes you feel like it's not a chore but a treat, going on walks can be a great form of exercise to improve your general wellbeing.

Endurance

If you're new to exercise or just have low stamina, walking can improve your physical endurance slowly, but surely. It's better to approach improving endurance that way, especially if you haven't done much exercise before. First, you might find it hard to walk a mile or so, for example. However, with a consistent and optimistic approach, you'll start to notice that it becomes easier and easier to go that distance.

Many people have trouble with exercise because they feel like it's a drag or a punishment. If you enjoy walking, you'll look forward to the time you get to spend doing so. You might not even notice all the progress you're making, because walking will start to feel so natural. If you want to get into other exercises, walking is an easy and effective gateway because it builds a good base for the higher endurance you'll need for more intense exercises.

Low Injury Risk

The low risk of injury that walking generally has is another positive. This is more a physical benefit in that in the long run, you probably won't have as many injuries as if you did something like martial arts or tackle football. Unless you're walking on high, jagged cliffs or through spiny forests, you'll probably have little to no chance of getting an injury. Walking is low-impact if done correctly (walk heel-toe!), and can be very relaxing.

Endorphins

As proven by countless studies, any form of exercise will release endorphins, whether it's just from one bout of exercise or more consistently over a longer period of time with consistent exercise. Walking isn't exempt from this rule, no matter how gentle the exercise may be. When you walk you release chemicals like adrenaline, dopamine, and other chemicals that create feelings of happiness in the brain.

Unlike when you eat your favorite dessert or watch a movie, the feelings aren't short-lasting. Of course, they'll go away eventually after you walk or do other exercises, but over time you'll build up a generally better base level of contentment with consistent exercise. This rule isn't necessarily foolproof should you have something like severe depression, but it can certainly aid in combating it.

Distraction

On one side of the mental benefits of walking is its use as a distraction. If you're having problems in life and need an escape or can't be alone with your own thoughts, walking is a good band-aid until you can get the help you need otherwise. For example, if you're depressed or anxious, putting in headphones and listening to your favorite podcast or album while taking a walk can calm your mental breakdown.

If possible, don't use it as the only salve to your mental health or life problems, as escapism isn't the best way to do things. It's best to get proper help. However, exercise is always positive, and can be a good way to tide yourself over until you have the resources or opportunities to get the help that you need. Even if your problems aren't that serious, it can be a good way to decompress or calm down.

Meditation

On the flip side of distracting yourself comes meditation. Most people are familiar with the idea of seated meditations, but walking can also provide a meditative state for some. Even in more loose terms, walking is a positive way to do something repetitively. This repetition can lead some to a state of focusing more clearly on their thoughts, which can lead to them working out any problems they may have been considering. What's equally possible is that the person walking may have thoughts and issues come to light that they never even considered possible, but their subconscious issues start to come to light. Some people say that walking is a form of therapy, and this may be why.

In its more literal sense, to do a walking meditation requires mindfulness. Like a seated mindful meditation, you need to focus on the sensations of walking, breathing, and other processes that normally would seem to be second nature. You let your thoughts fly by without judgment or criticism, and focus on picking your foot up, moving it forward, placing it down, doing the same with the other foot, and taking breaths in and out. For those who want to meditate but feel unable to when sitting down, this can serve as a more active alternative.

Walking is one of the best ways for releasing tension, both physical and mental. It can improve one's stamina, their mental state, and prove as a gateway for other exercises. It's a low-risk and low-impact exercise, but it's one of the most beneficial ones out there. If you're just getting into exercise or want to get into walking, you should start today!

TIP #12: SIX EXERCISES TO BUILD MUSCLE AT HOME

A gym is a great way to build muscle. However, gyms are not a requirement for becoming stronger. You can certainly build plenty of muscle while working out from home, especially if you are a newcomer to strength training. Here are six of the best exercises to perform at home to increase your muscles mass.

1. Push-ups.
This classic exercise is one of the foundations of bodyweight fitness. Push-ups primarily target the chest (pectorals) and arm (triceps) muscles while also requiring stomach and back muscles to be activated. Regularly doing push-ups plays a key role in beginning to grow muscle. Once standard push-ups become a little easier, graduate to more demanding, advanced variants such as decline, diamond, or even one-arm push-ups.

2. Squats.
Squats are another basic element of bodyweight fitness. This simple exercise -- which can even be performed while watching TV -- works virtually every major muscle in the lower half of the body, from the calves, to the quadriceps, hamstrings, and glutes. Squats also target the muscles found in the core to a smaller extent.

3. Planks.
This basic exercise is one of the essential parts of any fitness routine that eschews complicated equipment. While simple to perform, planks are nonetheless still demanding. Even people in great shape can benefit a lot from planks. There are also a huge number of plank variations that will force the body to work in

different ways.

4. Lunges.

Doing lunges is a great way to strengthen your glute, hamstring, and quadriceps muscles. Performing a single lunge isn't particularly difficult, but with further reps the exercise becomes much more challenging. Lunge variants, such as the lateral lunge or walking lunge, can be used to add more challenge as well.

5. Dips.

While dips can be completed using gym equipment, performing at-home variants using a chair is also perfectly possible. Dips are a compound exercise, which means they involve multiple joints and muscle groups. A fantastic upper body exercise, dips target the pectorals, deltoids, triceps, and abdominal muscles all at once.

6. Curls.

Curls are perfect for increasing arm strength and building the biceps. While most of the at home exercises to grow muscle require no equipment, performing curls does mean you will need some dumbbells. Luckily, dumbbells are not expensive when considering how useful they can be. Besides curls, dumbbells can also be used to make exercises like squats and lunges more challenging.

Strength training at home does have its drawbacks. Without the equipment found in a gym, your ability to grow muscle is ultimately limited. Past a certain point you will require the serious resistance provided by gym equipment if you wish to continue making progress. Still, growing your muscle with simple home workouts is certainly possible, and is a great way for an inexperienced person to introduce themselves to the habit of strength training.

TIP #13: SIX REASONS TO HIRE A PERSONAL TRAINER

Thousands of people every year vow to get into shape; some achieve their goals, while some don't quite get there. The people who do make exercise a part of their lifestyles may eventually run into a wall and need some help to start seeing progress again. For the people who don't quite make it, a little bit of motivation and accountability may have been all they needed to push through. A personal trainer is someone who could help in these situations. If you have never considered hiring a personal trainer before, here are six reasons that may change your mind.

You Are New to Fitness
Just like in any new venture, fitness can be intimidating. The gym can be an incredibly intimidating environment. Even if you manage to figure out the equipment, where do you start?

A personal trainer can help get you going in the right direction. Your trainer should perform assessments that will help to build the right program for you. These assessments will not only include your fitness levels, but take into account your lifestyle as well. The goal of the trainer should be to get you to the point of enjoying exercise so that it becomes a lifetime endeavor.

You Have Stopped Seeing Results
When you start a new exercise program, you will see results. The body is adjusting to the input it is getting, and it will respond accordingly by beginning to lose extra pounds and get stronger. You will start to see the health benefits of exercise. However, the human body is marvelous, and it will soon adapt to what you are doing. The body will adjust to this new normal, so you will need

to shake it up.

Personal trainers are experienced in all types of exercises and techniques. They can look at your routine with a fresh set of eyes and make adjustments to get your body to respond once again. Trainers can build a program that will vary your exercise routines, providing the results you want by keeping your body guessing.

You Need a Shakeup in Your Routine

If exercise isn't fun, it soon becomes a burden. Activity is something you'll want to do for the rest of your life. It would help if you had an inventory of different routines and exercises that keep you coming back for more. A personal trainer is an excellent resource to tap into for new ideas.

You Need a Challenge

Over time, even if you keep your exercise routines fun and exciting, you may want a little more out of your exercise program. As you begin to get into better shape, you will need to keep challenging your body to get the most out of your exercise time. Hire a trainer to help bring that challenge back to your workout program.

You Need Accountability

Repetition is the key to building lasting habits. However, sometimes willpower isn't enough to keep you going. It would be best if you had that little extra push and motivation that a personal trainer can provide. You're less likely to turn off that alarm, rollover, and go back to sleep if you know someone is waiting for you. Use your trainer as that accountability partner. Not to mention that you are paying them!

You Need Support

Sometimes you need a word of motivation to get through a challenging workout. Someone to listen to how sore you are would be nice too. Personal trainers are not only there for technical advice; they are also there as a support system. They are the sympathetic ear for you. They will be that cheerleader for you. Your trainer should have your best interests at heart and want to see you succeed.

These are just six of the many reasons that hiring a personal trainer is an excellent decision to make in your fitness journey. Your gym might already have a personal trainer on staff that you can use. If not, usually an internet search can turn up reputable trainers. Personal trainers most likely are in the profession because of their need to help people. You don't have to be on this journey all on your own.

TIP #14: FIVE CARDIO EXERCISES THAT HELP YOU BURN FAT FAST

There is no better way to burn fat than high-intensity cardio workouts. While cardio can be intimidating to a beginner who is trying to get fit, there are a variety of different cardio routines you can try. Whatever your exercise preferences, there is most certainly a cardio workout that fits your needs.

1. Running

Running is a classic cardio exercise and for good reason. Running burns a lot of calories and increases the strength of your heart without causing a burning sensation in your muscles. If you hate the sting in your legs while you bike, running may insure you can do cardio for a longer period of time without discomfort. If you're significantly overweight, running might not be the best option for you as it's high-impact, and injuries while running are fairly common.

2. Jump Rope

Jumping rope is an excellent way to get your heart racing fast without having to deal with the tedious feeling that running gives you. If you're someone who struggles to work out because you find it boring, jumping rope is a fun way to get your cardio in and burn some fat. The best part is that jumping rope is cheap. Jump ropes do not cost much and you can do it anywhere, no gym membership required.

3. Swimming

If you struggle with cardio because of an injury or body weight, consider swimming. If you're overweight, swimming will reduce the effects of gravity while still strengthening your heart.

It's not easy to swim laps, as you'll soon find out. But you'll be able to do it successfully regardless of weight or past injuries. Swimming is low-impact and you don't have to worry about hurting your body while in the pool. Even floating in water after doing a few laps is a great way for a beginner to burn calories.

4. Rowing Machine

If you want to gain muscle while you do your cardio routine, the rowing machine will be perfect for you. A rowing machine works out all the muscle groups in your body at one time, including your heart. It's not unrealistic to burn 1,000 calories an hour using a rowing machine because it requires so much effort from your body. The rowing machine might wear you out and you may struggle with it in the beginning, but you'll be rewarded in time with a toned physique.

5. Biking

Whether you bike outdoors or use a stationary bike at the gym, cycling is a great cardio workout to burn calories. Similar to swimming, it's low impact and you have minimal opportunity to injure yourself on a stationary bike. Unlike running, you'll feel more of a burn in your legs as biking helps to build your leg muscles. If you have limited time to bike, high intensity interval training will insure you burn fat as quickly as possible.

Cardio doesn't have to be a draining task. If you try several different types of cardio, you'll likely find there is a cardio workout that you actually enjoy. Choose the exercise you find most fun and burn off those calories.

TIP #15: FIVE SIGNS YOU NEED TO CHANGE YOUR EXERCISE ROUTINE

Have you been doing the same exercise routine for months and no longer feel like your current workout serves you or gives you the results you're looking for? If that's the case, it might be time to make a few changes to your workout or give it a total reboot. Change can help you better reach your objectives and stay motivated too.

You No Longer Feel the Challenge

Exercise shouldn't feel too easy unless you're doing it to relax. If you're trying to get results, you need some challenge. When you start working out, your body isn't accustomed to the movements you're doing. The exercises feel like a challenge and this forces your muscles to adapt and become stronger. But if you keep doing the same movements in the same way, the movements begin to feel easier. That's because you've become stronger or developed greater endurance. At that point, you need to work your muscles a little harder to continue to make gains. That's why using progressive overload (adding more weight, volume, or using more advanced techniques) is so important. It gives your muscles a new stimulus and challenge that causes them to further adapt. Even if you use progressive overload, there may come a point where you need to add different exercises or change your workout to make it challenging again.

Your Heart Rate Isn't Rising Enough

When you first launch into an aerobic training program, you might notice that your heart rate climbs quickly to the point where you get cardiovascular benefits. But if you keep doing the same routine at the same intensity, your heart rate doesn't rise as much during a workout. That's because your heart has become a more efficient pump and your cardiovascular fitness has improved. On the downside, unless you add more intensity, it will be hard to make further gains in aerobic fitness. Therefore, you must up the intensity of your training sessions. If you run or cycle, pick up the pace and add some hills, but be sure to track your heart rate to see how your cardiovascular system responds to these changes.

You're No Longer Getting Results

It's not uncommon for people to lift weights for a while and see changes in the beginning. In response to training, they become stronger and their muscles increase in size. But sometimes those changes come to a complete stop after a few months. You're frustrated to find that you're no longer experiencing gains in strength or changes in body composition. If that's the case, it's time to make your routine more challenging by lifting heavier weights, by increasing the number of repetitions, or by adding more sets. You can also introduce more advanced training techniques like supersets to challenge your muscles in a different way.

You Don't Feel as Motivated

Lack of motivation is a sign you need to change your exercise routine too, if only to fire yourself up again. If you've lost the passion, you won't give your workouts your best shot and won't be as successful in the long run. If you're skipping more and more workouts because you aren't as excited about your workout as you used to be, it's time to make some changes!

Are you bored with the type of workout you're doing or do you simply not feel challenged anymore? If the latter is the case, you may only need to increase the intensity of your current workout so you feel more challenged. If the added intensity doesn't help you get your mojo back, it may be time to completely change your approach. For example, you could take a break from lifting dumbbells and switch to barbells, resistance bands, or do body-weight exercises. You could also add new exercises to your routine. Sometimes changing only a few exercises is enough to re-ignite your passion for exercise and give you new motivation.

You Have Different Goals

Sometimes you need to change your workout because your goals have changed. For example, you lifted heavy weights for months to get stronger and now you'd like to lose body fat and get leaner. In that case, you could replace a portion of your heavy strength lifts with high-intensity interval training or moderate-intensity cardio to burn more calories. When your goals change, so should your workouts. That's the beauty of exercising: there are so many ways to do it and so many paths to getting fitter and stronger.

The Bottom Line

Don't let yourself get too locked into a workout that you're unwilling to make minor changes or completely redo your workout. Keep a fitness journal so you can track your goals and results and see whether you're meeting them or slowing down. You might also need to change your fitness routine if your current workout becomes mentally stale. Otherwise, your brain will help you find excuses not to work out.

TIP #16: DON'T FEEL LIKE EXERCISING TODAY? HERE'S WHY YOU SHOULD DO IT ANYWAY

If you're like most people, you have days when you just don't want to exercise. You've had a long day and are already tired after a day of too much work and not enough relaxation. Not only are you fatigued but you're in a crabby mood and feeling a bit down or under the weather. On days when you're not feeling motivated, it's tempting to throw in the towel and take the day off and relax in front of the television or with a good book in your lap. You can always make up for it when you do your next workout, right?

Unless you're sick or sleep-deprived, there are important reasons to do your workout anyway. Why should you reconsider your decision not to exercise? Research shows that exercise is a mood booster. According to Harvard Health and a study published in JAMA psychiatry, the odds of feeling depressed dropped by 26% with each significant increase in physical activity. Working out helps chase away boredom, and there's a physiological basis for how exercise fights depression.

Studies show that a vigorous workout boosts endorphins, natural chemicals that relieve pain and lift mood. Researchers believe endorphins play a role in the runner's high, the feeling of well-being and calmness that people experience during and after a run. Research even shows that exercise boosts creativity and can help you come up with new ideas and fresh solutions to problems. In some ways, it's like a reboot for your body and brain.

What about your fatigue and lack of motivation? It's hard to lace up your exercise shoes and launch into a workout when you're fatigued, but research shows exercise can boost your energy level. Once you get going and blood and oxygen begins pulsing to every cell in your body, it lifts your spirits and your energy level.

One study found that people who said they dreaded taking a walk and thought it wouldn't make them feel better reported feeling more energetic, positive, alert, and confident afterward. Sometimes it's best not to listen to those negative voices that tell you that you're too tired to move your body and push through anyway.

Flex Your Self-Discipline Muscle
Another reason to exercise on days you don't feel like it is it re-inforces self-discipline. Motivation isn't the most important factor for long-term exercise success; it's self-discipline. Motivation is short-term and often based on emotion, while self-discipline keeps you going after the initial flush of excitement of starting an exercise program dies down.

When you exercise on days you don't want to, you flex your self-discipline muscle and make it stronger. When you don't succumb to excuses not to exercise, it becomes easier to stay on track in the future. You're telling your body that it's okay to be tired, but there's still work to do and a plan to follow. After all, you can't call into work every time you feel tired, right? How much more successful people would be with exercise training if they treated it with the reverence they treat their job. Exercising when you don't want to keeps your self-discipline muscle from getting flabby.

How to Exercise When You Don't Feel Like It
Sometimes granting permission not to exercise hard will help you follow through on days when you don't want to do it. Tell

yourself you'll exercise for only 10 minutes. After 10 minutes are up, you have permission to stop. Almost anyone can do something for 10 minutes. Once 10 minutes elapse, there's a good chance you'll keep going. Once your body adapts to the shock of movement, you'll feel better and you probably won't mind continuing. It's the initial inactivity that's so intimidating.

Think back to days you didn't exercise. How did you feel on those days? Chances are, you felt less energetic and maybe experienced a little guilt that you sat so much and didn't get your body moving. Keep that in mind when you don't feel like exercising too. Knowing the positive things that exercise does for your mental and physical health is extra motivation when you feel tired.

Know When Not to Exercise Too

This doesn't mean you should always work out when you don't feel well. If you only slept two hours the night before, you feel like you're getting sick, or already have an illness, it would be foolish to push your body too hard. Don't exercise if you have a fever or if you have symptoms that extend below your neck, such as a cough. Be sensible and don't harm your mental or physical health by exercising when you truly aren't up for it, but don't be too easy on yourself either.

The Bottom Line

Not only can exercise boost your mood and give you more energy on those days that you feel tired, pushing through strengthens self-discipline, so you'll be more capable of sticking with your plan to get into and stay in shape. Keep the longer-term goal in mind. If you constantly find reasons to not work out, you'll eventually give up in frustration.

If you find you're questioning whether to work out too often, change the time you're working out. Of course, you're tired after a long day at work. Why not exercise first thing in the morning while you're still fresh? Choose the path with less resistance that still allows you to stay on track, and the next time your body tells you that you're too tired, cover your ears!

TIP #17: HOME EXERCISE EQUIPMENT YOU CAN BUY TO AVOID GYM MEMBERSHIP

Taking time out of your day to drive to the gym simply isn't easy for a busy lifestyle. Whether you live far away from your local gym or simply don't have extra time in your schedule, getting home exercise equipment may be the right decision for you. Don't let the difficulty of getting to a gym daily keep you from reaching your fitness goals. Choose any of the following pieces of exercise equipment to start a convenient work out routine at home.

1. Treadmill

A treadmill requires a fair amount of space in your home but is the perfect piece of home exercise equipment if you enjoy running. Living in a hot climate can hinder your ability to run outside during the summer. Likewise, if you live where it snows it can be unsafe to run during the winter. With a treadmill, you can run regardless of the weather patterns outside. Running on a treadmill will also limit leg and knee injuries as it's significantly easier on your body than running on concrete or asphalt. As long as you've got the room and the money for a treadmill, it's a solid piece of exercise equipment.

2. Stationary Bike

Biking is a fantastic way to get low-impact cardio workout. Biking causes less strain and injury on your body than running does but will still get your heart rate up. A stationary bike is an excellent choice if you have limited space for equipment as you can find folding bikes that can be easily stored away. An exercise bike is significantly cheaper than a treadmill so if you're looking for affordable cardio equipment, a bike may be perfect for you.

3. Rowing Machine

A rowing machine is one of the only pieces of exercise equipment that exercises every muscle group in the body while also providing a healthy cardio workout. If you're looking for a piece of equipment for both cardio and strength training, look no further than a rowing machine. Rowing machines come in a wide range of prices, do your research and figure out what machine best fits your budget and needs.

4. Punching Bag

A punching bag can provide a great arm and cardio workout if you use it correctly. Many people who don't enjoy traditional cardio find that a punching bag provides a more fun way to exercise. You might forget how long you've been working out as you punch away. A punching bag will be especially beneficial for anyone with an interest in boxing or martial arts

5. Elliptical Machine

Similar to a treadmill, an elliptical machine will require a lot of space and can be fairly expensive. But the benefits of an elliptical machine are numerous. You can increase both your strength and stamina with this cardio work out. If you find running exhausting, you may find an elliptical machine more enjoyable. You can strength train your legs and reach your target heart rate on an elliptical machine.

Which piece of exercise equipment best fits your home and fitness goals is entirely up to you. Choose the piece of equipment that best accommodates your space and budget. Utilizing any of the above pieces of gym equipment at home will make it significantly easier to attain a healthy exercise routine.

TIP #18: SURPRISE! EVEN A TWO MINUTE WORKOUT CAN BENEFIT YOUR HEART

Despite the many health benefits of exercise, few people work out consistently. The reason? Many people cite a lack of time. However, the time you devote to doing it is a good investment when you consider the health benefits. The current guidelines recommend getting 150 minutes of moderate-intensity exercise or 75 minutes of high-intensity exercise each week.

Well, what if you could get the health benefits of exercise by working out only two minutes? Does it sound too good to be true? It's not. Research shows that 120 seconds of exercise could offer similar benefits at the cellular level to exercising for 30 minutes or more, at a significant time savings.

If You Work Out Less, Intensity Matters
The downside of a 2-minute workout is that it can't be leisurely. In other words, you can't take a stroll around your house for 2 minutes and expect your cardiovascular health to improve. You will get points for not sitting, but it's not the equivalent to the benefits you'll get from exercising more intensely.

During a 2-minute workout, you must work hard enough to sweat and feel challenged to keep going. Imagine sprinting across a field as opposed to taking a leisurely jog. You could also get a 2-minute workout by jumping rope at a fast pace for 2 minutes. However, the easiest way to do a short workout is through high-intensity interval training.

How effective is it? In a study, researchers asked participants to ride an exercise bike at 50% of their maximum intensity for 30 minutes. At such an intensity, you're pedaling at a relatively comfortable pace. Another group cycled for 4 minutes at 75% of their maximum effort. This group did this 5 times in a row for 20 minutes. The final group did four intense pedaling sessions on an exercise bike for 30 seconds at a time. In between each session, they rested for 4.5 minutes. So, the latter group only exerted for a total of 2 minutes excluding the rest periods between each active session. This is similar to what people do when they interval train.

The results? The group who exerted themselves for only 2 minutes experienced similar changes at the cellular level as the group who worked out at a moderate intensity for 30 minutes.

What were these changes? Inside cells are tiny organelles called mitochondria. Their job is to produce the energy currency, called ATP, that all cells use to do work. Every time your muscles contract, they require ATP to make it possible. Without it, all movement would come to a standstill. When your cells have more mitochondria, you have better exercise endurance. Plus, research links more mitochondria with better heart health.

Having more mitochondria is beneficial for metabolic health, too. Aging mitochondria are a cause of insulin resistance, where cells don't respond as well to insulin. This causes a rise in insulin that increases fat storage inside skeletal muscle. Over time, this increases the risk of type 2 diabetes and cardiovascular disease. Short bursts of exercise help keep the mitochondria inside cells healthy and plentiful. You also lose mitochondria because of aging and intense exercise, even in small amounts, helps stem this loss.

If you need more proof that short, intense periods of exercise work, a study found that only two weeks of high-intensity interval exercise increased the number and function of mitochondria inside muscle cells.

The Bottom Line

You can boost the number of mitochondria inside your cells with short bursts of exercise, as long as you keep the intensity high. In fact, the benefits are similar to what you get from 30 minutes of moderate-intensity exercise. Short, intense workouts are more manageable for time-challenged exercisers. However, it's best to ease into intense workouts. Build up a baseline level of fitness by walking briskly for 10 minutes at a time for a few weeks. Once you're conditioned, ease into short, high-intensity workouts.

You can choose any form of exercise for the active intervals, as long as you do it with intensity. Some people use an exercise bike or sprint, but you could also jump rope, use an elliptical machine, rowing machine, do plyometric jumps, or swing a kettlebell with intensity during the active intervals. You can vary the type of exercise you do during the active intervals too. The only condition is to work as hard as you can during the active intervals. Then, you get to rest. It's a time expedient way to enjoy the health benefits of exercise.

TIP #19: FIVE BENEFITS OF WARMING UP BEFORE EXERCISE AND WHY YOU SHOULD NOT SKIP IT

Do you think warming up before exercise is a waste of time? Many people want to get to the "meat" of the workout and skip the groundwork. As a result, they either skip it or do a super fast and sloppy warm-up. If you're doing it right, a warm-up should last around 10 minutes. It takes that much time to get the blood flowing to all of your muscles and your muscles primed to work. So don't skip it. Here are five reasons you need a warm-up every time you work out:

Warming Up Gets You Mentally Primed

Half the battle of getting into shape is having the right mindset. A 10-minute warm-up offers a chance to review in your mind your upcoming workout, your goals, and how you'll accomplish them. In other words, it gets your head in the right place. Don't underestimate how important that is! Your mind is more power-ful than you think. A study found that people who envisioned doing biceps curls in their minds gained strength even though they never touched a weight. It's not just what your muscles do that count; it's what goes on in your head too. Spend warm-up time focusing on the upcoming exercises.

A Warm-Up is Safer for Your Cardiovascular System

If you suddenly broke into a run from a standing or sitting posi-tion, your heart would have to speed up quickly Such demands place added stress on your heart and blood vessels. That's why a warm-up is so important. A thorough warm-up is especially important if you have high blood pressure, type 2 diabetes, or a heart problem. Of course, you should always get clearance from your physician if you have health issues before starting to work out.

Warming Up Improves Muscle Flexibility

Another benefit of a warm-up is it increases your core body temperature. As your body temperature rises, it warms your muscles and tendons and increases muscle flexibility and elasticity. Cold, stiff muscles are more likely to develop strains or tears. So, warming up could help you avoid a painful strain or injury. If you don't feel like warming up, just remember how inconvenient it is to injure yourself and not be able to work out. If you work out first thing in the morning, lengthen your warm-up a bit since your muscles will be cold and stiff after 8 hours of inactivity.

A Warm-Up Prepares Your Muscles for Working Together

Another benefit of a warm-up is, by engaging the nervous system and muscles, it improves communication between the two systems. Your nervous system tells your muscles to contract and "calls the shots." Warming up with dynamic movements wakes up your muscles and nervous system and gets them ready to work together as a team. This leads to safer and better performance.

Warming Up Can Improve Your Performance

Whether you're doing a resistance training workout or a high-intensity interval session, a warm-up increases muscle elasticity. More elastic muscles enhance your range-of-motion when you do certain exercises. An analysis of 32 studies published in the Journal of Strength and Conditioning Research that looked at a variety of performance criteria found warming up improved 79% of them. Plus, they found that warming up had no downsides. This analysis has credibility because it looked at so many criteria and studies and pooled the results.

What Should a Warm-Up Consist Of?

A warm-up should include 5 to 10 minutes of light exercise that targets the upper and lower body. Good warm-up exercises include light jogging, jumping jacks, arm swings, leg swings, kicks, punches, or lateral shuffles. Feel free to do a variety of these movements. Don't push it! The goal is to incrementally increase your heart rate and blood flow to the muscles. Start at a very slow pace and gradually boost the intensity, but you shouldn't be huffing and puffing. No need to tire yourself out before the real work begins. Once you've completed your warm-up, you're ready to start the meat of the workout.

The Bottom Line

The warm-up might seem like a waste of time or something that steals time from the main production but it has an important purpose, to get your body and mind prepared for exercise. Doing one may even help your performance and lower your risk of injury. If you're in a hurry, you can cut a few minutes off of your warm-up, but a warm-up should be at least 5 minutes. Now you know why warming up matters. Use it to your advantage.

TIP #20: FOUR BENEFITS OF REGULAR EXERCISE

Do you ever drive past the gym and wonder if working out is really worth the effort?. It's only natural for you to wonder what it gives you in return. A lean or muscular body is an obvious benefit, but does exercising offer anything else? The answer is yes. Below you'll find four incredible benefits you'll experience if you make exercise part of your weekly routine.

Exercise Helps Control Your Weight
Weight control is a well known benefit, but it's still worth talking about. Many Americans complain about extra pounds that they'd like to lose. Several people have tried crash dieting or drinking special mixtures as a cleanse. These extremes may produce results, but they're not lasting. If you lose weight simply by dieting, the moment you reach your goal and begin eating outside the parameters of that diet, you'll start to add the weight back. Gaining weight after working so hard, simply because you 'splurged' is what destroys motivation in so many. Dieters can't understand why they can't keep the weight off.

The reason is, you have nothing burning the added calories you've put back into your diet. Losing weight should be done by dieting and working out. When you combine diet and exercise, it not only helps you lose weight, but it controls your weight and helps you keep it off. As you exercise and gain muscle, every pound of muscle you gain burns around 6.5 calories an hour without any added effort from you. Your added muscle, and the calories it burns, will help balance everything out when you stop your strict diet upon reaching your goal. Plus, during the weight loss process, exercise will help you to burn fat faster, helping you reach your goals in a shorter time frame.

Exercise Helps Lower Your Risk for Certain Health Conditions
Everyone wants to live longer, be happier, and feel good inside their own bodies. There's no miracle drug that will help you achieve all of that, but exercise can. Exercise helps your body to function as if it were younger than it actually is, much like excess fat and unhealthy eating will make your body function as if it were older.

Exercise also boosts your HDL levels (Healthy Cholesterol) and simultaneously lowers your LDL levels (Unhealthy Cholesterol). This combination radically improves your heart health and decreases your risk of cardiovascular diseases. Staying active by exercising regularly will also help prevent stroke, type 2 diabetes, a number of cancers, and arthritis. It is a health boost unlike any other, making it one of the best decisions you can make for your body and overall health.

Exercise Improves Your Mood
Not only does exercise help your body look and feel better, but it also helps improve your mental health and emotional levels. Physical activity like running, biking, or a Zumba class can help stimulate and release endorphins (feel-good chemicals) in your brain. Exercising not only releases good chemicals into your brain, it also reduces certain immune system chemicals that can worsen depression.

Regular exercise is often suggested for people with anxiety, high stress levels, or depression to help ease their symptoms and give them a much-needed boost of happiness and relaxation. Even if you're a generally happy person, but you've been stressed from a long week, exercising can benefit you in the same way. It will help improve your mood and give you a feeling of accomplishment along the way.

Exercise Boosts Your Energy

Exercising is exhausting when you first start, but over time it can actually increase your energy, strength, and endurance. You'll notice these improvements appear in stages. Lifting heavy objects will become easier, the workout routine that used to exhaust you doesn't seem as hard, vacuuming the house doesn't seem as daunting, and mowing the yard no longer requires a nap afterward. As you continue to make exercise a regular part of your routine, you'll notice your physical limitations being pushed further and further away.

Exercise may seem like a chore at first, but the more you do it, the more you'll love it. There's something empowering about tackling a challenge and then rising to a new one. As you continue to physically push yourself, you'll notice you feel better, look better, and have more confidence. Exercise offers truly life-changing results if you're willing to put in the effort required.

TIP #21: FIVE WAYS STRENGTH TRAINING SLOWS AGING

You know strength training benefits your body composition and improves the way you look, but did you know working your muscles against resistance also slows aging? If there's one thing all humans want, it's to be fit and functional as long as possible. Strength training can help you be your healthiest self and even slow the aging process, but have you ever wondered how? Here are five ways strength training helps you stay more youthful and why it's a good investment.

Strength Training Prevents Muscle Loss Due to Aging
Most people begin to lose muscle mass during the middle of the third decade of life. The rate of muscle loss is faster and more pronounced in people who aren't active. Strength training slows muscle loss, so much so that people who strength train regularly often have the muscle composition of someone decades younger. You don't have to use barbells or dumbbells to get the benefits. Bodyweight exercises, such as push-ups, and resistance bands, are effective too and they're less intimidating when you first start out.

Strength Training Reduces Bone Loss Too
Osteoporosis is one of the leading health problems women face with age. In fact, one out of two women over the age of 50 will break a bone because of osteoporosis. You start losing bone during the second to third decade of life and bone loss speeds up after menopause. Women who are small-boned or thin are at higher risk, and smoking also increases the likelihood of devel-

oping osteoporosis.

Fortunately, strength training is healthy for your bones. When you work your muscles against resistance by lifting weight or doing bodyweight exercises, it pulls on the underlying bones. This action stimulates the laydown of new bone by bone-producing cells called osteoblasts. In turn, this reduces bone loss due to aging. Research suggests that lifting heavy weights (around 80% of one-rep max or greater) is most effective for stimulating the laydown of new bone, but some studies also suggest that using lighter weights and performing higher reps have some benefit too. The key is to fatigue the muscles you're working when you train.

The earlier you start training your muscles and bones against resistance, the better. You have the most bone mass in your mid-20s and it declines after that. Strength training slows this process down and helps lower the risk of osteoporosis.

Better Functionality
One of the most important reasons to strength train is to stay functional as the decades go by. What good is it to be alive if you struggle to do the things you enjoy? Strong muscles give you the ability to carry out the activities you do every day from keeping the house clean to enjoying a day at the beach. The old saying is right; if you don't use it, you'll lose it.

Using a fast tempo when you do some weight training sets is beneficial too. Moving a weight through space quickly builds muscle power, the ability to generate force quickly. That's important for functional activities, like getting up out of a chair. One reason older people end up in a wheelchair is that they don't have enough muscle power to thrust themselves up from a sitting position. Keep doing the things you enjoy for longer by working your body against resistance.

Strength Training Improves Metabolic Health

Cardiovascular disease and type 2 diabetes are two of the biggest health problems that shorten lifespans and speed up aging. Strength training improves how cells respond to insulin (insulin sensitivity), thereby improving blood sugar control. Training your muscles against resistance also helps with weight loss and weight control. Maintaining a healthy body weight and healthy insulin sensitivity lowers your risk of developing cardiovascular disease and type 2 diabetes. It's one of the many benefits of working your muscles against resistance.

Greater Longevity

This would be the biggest benefit of all! Believe it or not, research shows that being physically stronger could help you live longer, and getting that way won't happen by sitting on the couch. Studies where researchers measure muscle strength and follow those participants show that older adults who are stronger have up to a 50% lower risk of dying early. Other research looking at handgrip strength, for example, also shows a correlation between grip strength and reduced mortality.

The Bottom Line

Strength training gives you a healthier, more aesthetically pleasing physique but it can also slow the aging process and help you stay functional longer. Start where you are and at your own pace but take advantage of all the health and fitness benefits strength training offers.

TIP #22: SIX REASONS FOR FEELING UNUSUALLY TIRED DURING EXERCISE

Feeling tired is a normal part of exercise. In fact, it is often a sign of a great workout. However, there are different kinds of tiredness. If you are feeling completely drained just a few minutes into a workout, or are getting exhausted by exercises that used to be easy, there might be an underlying problem. Here are the six most likely causes.

1. Dehydration. Water is necessary for healthy bodily function during exercise. Lack of fluids reduces blood volume, making it harder for the heart to supply the muscles with the oxygen they need, resulting in exhaustion. Water is also needed for sweat, which is the means by which the body cools itself. Fight dehydration by drinking water regularly throughout the day, especially as your workout approaches. The general rule is to get six to eight glasses a day (more on hot days). Drinking water during a workout is also wise.

2. Insufficient recovery time. While exercise is incredibly good for you, it also puts a lot of strain on your body. It takes times for the body to bounce back from such stress. The harder a workout, the more recovery is required. An especially intense exercise session should be followed by days of easier work. Having variety in your workout routine is also crucial. Don't keep practicing the same kinds of exercise day after day. Mix it up by doing both cardio and strength training, and target different areas of the body.

3. Vitamin deficiency. Vitamins and minerals are vital for proper body functioning. While all vitamins and minerals are important, insufficient iron consumption is a particularly likely cause of lethargy. That's because iron is needed for the delivery of oxygen to the muscles. Deficiencies of vitamin D, vitamin B, copper, magnesium, and potassium can all cause trouble as well. In general, the solution to a vitamin or mineral deficiency is simply to eat a healthy, balanced diet -- meaning lots of fruits, vegetables, and healthy proteins, with a minimum of processed and fatty foods.

4. Lack of carbs. Carbohydrates often get a bad rap. However, while it can be good to limit carb consumption, they are not bad for you -- especially when it comes to working out. That's because exercise burns a lot of energy. The main source for energy is glucose, which is primarily derived from carbs. Consuming too few carbohydrates means exhaustion, especially during aerobic workouts. To maintain a good diet, opt for healthier carbs such as whole grains.

5. Medications. Many kinds of medications can cause tiredness, including both over-the-counter and prescription drugs. Among the potential culprits are antihistamines, used to treat allergies and colds. Antidepressants and anti-anxiety drugs can cause lethargy too. Beta-blockers, which lower blood pressure, can also result in the muscles getting insufficient blood supply. Statins, which treat high cholesterol, can disrupt normal energy production. Of course, you can't stop taking an important medicine simply because it makes exercise difficult. Instead, ask your doctor if there is an alternative.

6. Poor sleep. In light of how few people in today's world sleep well, bad sleep might be the biggest cause of tiredness during exercise. Sleep is when the body recovers from the strains (both physical and mental) of life. Thus it is impossible to feel refreshed and energetic without quality sleep. Bad sleep means your body is likely not even fully recovered from your last workout. Aim for eight solid hours a night. Promote better sleep by following a regular sleep schedule, shutting down electronics close to bedtime, and minimizing stress.

The occasional workout off-day is to be expected, and is not a cause for concern. But if you are having more trouble, you need to address the problem. Most of the potential causes of exhaustion outlined above are serious matters that shouldn't be ignored. If your issues with lethargy during exercise persist, visit a medical professional.

TIP #23: SHOULD I TAKE A BREAK FROM WORKING OUT?

Fitness devotees know that the key to long-term health and fitness is to exercise at least five times a week, if not daily. A fitness regimen is the best way to stay healthy, prevent disease, reduce stress, and live longer. However, there are days when you just aren't feeling it, or maybe an illness has left you bedridden for a week. Work schedules and family life can also be extremely demanding, leaving you drained of the energy needed to work out. And you're probably wondering if you do take breaks, will you lose your fitness gains? How long is too long to take a break from exercise, and can I regain my previous fitness level?

Taking a break

Whether you are taking a break because you feel you need a rest or you are ill, you're probably worried about losing your strength and endurance. According to the American Council on Exercise, taking a break from working out (if you already work out 4-6 times a week) is good for the mind and body to rest and recover. Taking a full week off for someone who is already fit is positive and beneficial. You won't lose any strength or endurance, and you won't gain any weight. Recovery time allows your muscle tissues to regenerate and deliver nutrients to your body.

Yet, for most people, the battle is more mental than physical when they stop working out, especially beginners. According to Dr. Steve Bell from the University of Minnesota, newbies to exercise are most at risk of quitting their workout routine after a break. For beginners, getting out of the routine of exercise when just beginning may cause some people to quit exercising altogether.

The takeaway here is that regular exercisers are encouraged to take short breaks, as they will not lose any gains, while novices should not take a long break until their routine is established, as it may affect motivation.

Recovery and rest
Taking a break from your workout routine doesn't mean turning into a couch potato. You still need movement to stay healthy and keep blood circulating to your muscles. The American Council on Exercise defines recovery as removing strenuous exercise for a day or week--essentially a non-training day. If you feel you need a break but don't want to stop your momentum, taking a stroll or practicing restorative yoga is a great way to let your muscles recover while also allowing progress.

How long should recovery time be?
Recovery time is up to you and what your body needs. Listen to the signals your body is telling you. Are you sore? Feeling exhausted or overwhelmed? Take some time off if your body needs it. But the key here is, don't take too long of a break.

What happens when I stop working out?
Did you take the weekend off from your routine to rest this weekend? Don't worry, you haven't lost any gains--yet. For most people, it takes up to two months to lose the gains you've made overall. Aerobic and cardio fitness begins to decline faster, losing about 5-10% of aerobic fitness in about three weeks. Muscle endurance and strength last longer than aerobic fitness, however. For a regular person, this means you may begin to lose strength gains around two and a half to three weeks. Muscle memory helps retain strength up for a few weeks to even a few months, so you will lose endurance first before you notice a loss in strength gains.

Will I gain weight if I take a break?

The most dreaded aspect for most about taking a break from working out is gaining weight. Studies conducted at the University of Crete in Greece have shown that after a six-week break from exercise, most people will begin to gain weight and body fat, especially if they eat unhealthy, high- calorie foods. If you do decide to take an extended break, be sure to eat healthy, nutritious meals and keep up with calorie intake.

Workout routine alternatives

If you're feeling burnt out, fatigued, or you are injured, you still may not want to take a complete break from your workouts. Even if you are recovering, it is healthy and beneficial to still do low-impact, gentle exercises to keep your mind and body in shape. So if you don't feel like exercising strenuously, you could take a long walk, do gentle yoga, Pilates, tai chi, or even take a swim. During recovery days, incorporate gentle, low-impact exercises to help your muscles recover without causing further damage.

I took a long break from my workouts. How do I get back in shape?

If you have taken a long break from exercise, first check in with your doctor to get the all-clear to return to exercise, especially if you were ill. Take it slowly, and gently return to your routine. For instance, if you were jogging regularly, you might want to start back walking first, and if you lift weights, start at a lower weight and fewer reps. Allowing your body to gradually get accustomed to exercising again will help prevent injury, soreness, or fatigue. The idea is to start slowly so you can retrain your muscles and build your endurance.

The takeaway

Taking a break from working out has both pros and cons. Too long of a break and you risk gaining weight, losing muscle strength, endurance, and cardio fitness. Another risk of taking a break is losing your momentum and you might stop exercising altogether.

A short break, however, can be beneficial if your body needs it. A few days, or even up to a week off from your workouts can replenish your body, mind, and motivation. Like everything in life, find a good balance of both working out and rest to stay healthy.

TIP #24: HOW TO STAY ENERGIZED ALL DAY

Are you struggling to make your way through another sluggish day? Maybe you woke up exhausted, slumped your way through the morning, then felt like you were hit by a truck of bricks when the afternoon rolled around. You're not alone and you're not hopeless. Take these tips to get you going first thing in the morning and stay energized all day.

Start by Sleeping Well

Having the energy to excel from morning to evening begins the night before with a great night of sleep. Turn off your gadgets an hour before it's time to sleep, allow your body to decompress from the day, and go to bed in time to get the hours of rest necessary to feel rejuvenated for the next day.

Get up Early and Get Going

If you get to sleep at a reasonable hour, you're going to put yourself in a better position to wake up early and start your day before stressors begin to pounce. The extra time you'll have in the morning will allow you to use your time for more productive activities than those generally associated with late-night distractions.

Move Early, Move Often, and Get Some Sun

Now that you're rested and alert, start your day on the right track by getting outside, letting the sunlight prepare you for the rest of your day with a dose of vitamin D. Breathe in some fresh air and allow your body to wake up with exercise, whether it be a brisk walk or long-distance run. Keep your body moving throughout the day will help you take in more oxygen and keep your blood flowing efficiently.

Stay on Track with a Healthy Diet

Nothing will get you off course faster than energy crashing flurries of junk food, processed carbohydrate-loaded meals, and sugar-infused juice or soda. Your body reacts to what you eat, so consider maintaining a healthy diet that includes plenty of protein, complex carbohydrates, healthy fats, and a consistent intake of water to keep you hydrated.

Take a 10 Minute Power Nap

Not everyone can afford such a luxury, but if you're able to take a short nap in the afternoon, you'll feel better the rest of the day. Experts suggest that a 10-minute power nap can make you more alert and effective the rest of the day. If you're not in a place where a nap is prudent, at least make sure to take intermittent breaks from staring at electronics and let your body refresh.

Rock Some Tunes

Remember you're human with feelings and emotions that respond to outside stimuli. Find a playlist of music that gets you in the mood to make your days more productive. Similarly, you can reset your mind and body with a friendly conversation or another form of entertainment.

Rinse and Repeat

The most important step you will take to feel energized is when you decide to stick to a regular pattern of helpful behaviors. Anyone can have a slip-up, but if you determine to take action, you'll provide the best opportunities to stay energized all day, every day.

TIP #25: FIVE WAYS YOU'RE SABOTAGING YOUR EXERCISE ROUTINE

You know that exercise is good for you, but for one reason or another, it just isn't working out. Here are some ways that you might be sabotaging your exercise routine, as well as some suggestions for how to get back on the path to fitness success.

1. You put off exercising.
If you have too much to do and not enough time, it can be tempting to postpone exercise until you have some spare time - except that might never happen. Make exercise one of your top priorities. If you can't do it every day, try to work out at least three or four times per week, and create a regular slot in your schedule for it. If you exercise regularly, it will become a habit that will be hard to break.

2. Your exercise sessions are too long or too short.
A successful exercise routine follows the Goldilocks principle. It should be neither too long nor too short, but just right. If you don't exercise for long enough, you'll only gain minimal health benefits. However, if you push yourself too hard with a long, intense exercise session, you'll risk burnout and injury. The amount of time that you should spend exercising will depend on what type of exercise you're doing, your fitness goals and your physical condition. Consult a personal trainer or your health care provider to determine how long your exercise sessions should be.

3. You're exercising at the wrong time of the day.

Not only is it important to exercise for the right length of time, but it's also crucial to do it at the right time of the day. If you exercise within three hours of going to bed, you might find it hard to fall asleep. If you go jogging or do other types of intensive, cardiovascular exercise after a heavy meal, your stomach might rebel. There's not a single time of the day to exercise that will work for everyone, so find the right time for you. It might be in the morning, after you wake up, or in the evening after work, to recharge yourself. If you're not sure when your ideal time to exercise is, experiment with working out at different times of the day, and make a note of how you feel after each exercise session.

4. You're not having fun.

Exercise doesn't have to be dull and grueling. Forget those ideas of mindlessly pacing on a treadmill or doing endless repetitions of work outs. Instead, entertain yourself while you work out by listening to an interesting podcast or some lively music. Or, bring a friend to the gym, and chat while you sweat. Alternatively, you could ditch your old routine and try something new, such as enrolling in a fitness class or joining a local amateur sports team. If you search for fitness classes and sports that are offered in your community, you might be surprised at the variety of options you'll find.

5. You've given up.

Maybe you've decided that exercising is too hard, and you just can't do it anymore. Or, you've gotten bored or simply never started. Yes, exercise can be tough, especially when you're working out the kinks in a new routine, but the more you exercise, the easier it will be to stay motivated. You'll have "off" days, but if you keep it up, you'll notice progress over time. So, ignore all the self-doubt, and go for it! Consider seeking out a fitness buddy or personal trainer for moral support.

Exercising doesn't have to be difficult, boring and inconvenient. In fact, establishing a successful fitness routine might be easier than you think. Use these tips to help make each exercise session fun and productive.

TIP #26: HOW TO PUT ON TEN POUNDS OF MUSCLE

While much of the health industry is focused on weight loss, you might find yourself in need of some extra muscles, and it won't come by sitting on your couch. Take these steps to gain the extra muscle you need, starting today!

Start Compound Weight Lifting Immediately

If you want your muscles to grow, you're going to have to work for it; there is no other way. Implement compound weight lifting exercises that will challenge multiple muscles with every movement as you improve balance and coordination. You are going to need to put forth maximum intensity in your workout sessions, pushing your muscles to their limit, and increasing your efforts in subsequent days. Compound weight training exercises can be as simple as push-ups and squats or involve free weight exercises with dumbbells and barbells such as the bench press and deadlift.

Load Up on the Right Food

If you want your muscles to grow, you're going to need to feed yourself with the fuel it needs to function properly. It's time to eliminate junk food and sugar products. Replace them with lean proteins, such as chicken breasts and fish, as well as complex carbs such as whole grains, beans, and vegetables. Remember you're trying to grow, so pile on the extra calories, but keep them nutritious. If you have trouble getting enough food into your system, you can always add a powdered whey protein shake into the mix.

Recover! Get Rest and Sleep

Your body is more than a machine. You are a living being designed for alternating periods of work and rest. Since you want your muscles to grow, you need to not only exercise and feed them, but also give them time to repair and restructure the way you want them. Rest your muscles between workouts and get enough sleep at night so your body can do what it needs to do to gain those extra ten pounds of desired muscle.

Muscles won't grow without help, but if you take the necessary steps, they'll be more willing to cooperate with your goals. Do the right things consistently, including exercise, refueling, and recovery, and you'll see the growth you're looking for.

TIP #27: IS THIS WHY YOU SEE NO RESULTS WHEN YOU EXERCISE?

Whether you're an athlete or someone who hates to get off the sofa, there are a number of mistakes that you can make with your diet that can keep you from getting the most out of the exercise that you put in. Here are some of the most serious ways in which your diet misconceptions can affect your exercise plan.

Banishing all fat from your diet
Many exercise nutrition books are at pains to repeatedly remind people who exercise that they need healthy fats from nuts and seeds for good muscle growth and overall health. Even so, it's difficult for people to set aside the fear of fat that they've learned their whole lives.

Whether your aim is to lose weight or to become more powerful as an athlete, you need healthy fat in your diet. Fat is important for a number of reasons. If your aim is to lose weight, you need fats in your diet to feel filled up sooner and to keep from feeling hunger too often. Healthy fats also improve the way your body absorbs the antioxidants in the fruits and vegetables that you eat. New research indicates that packing one's diet with antioxidants helps the body stay lean. A good supply of fat also raises your body's basic metabolic rate – helping you burn calories more quickly.

If you are an athlete, you need fat in your diet to help in the process of muscle recovery. Fat is an important component of the basic structure of each cell in your body. Your cells need fat to repair themselves. Taking too much fat off your diet can result in fatigue and muscles that are prone to injury.

The lesson to learn here is clear – whether you need to lose weight or improve your performance as an athlete, you need enough healthy fats in your diet. Be sure to dress your salads in olive oil. You can use olive oil to sauté your vegetables, too.

Using sports drinks more than you need to

If the way you exercise makes you sweat heavily – perhaps you put yourself through intense workouts or you perform your workouts in hot and humid weather – staying hydrated with a sports drink is a smart decision. Sports drinks help put the electrolytes that you lose to sweating back in your body. If you don't sweat too much when you exercise, though (perhaps you get your workouts in an air-conditioned gym or perhaps you don't exercise more than a half hour at a time) a regular drink of plain water is all you need.

Choosing water over a sports drink isn't just about cutting unnecessary expense. Sports drinks are filled with sugar and carbohydrates. Knocking back a bottle of sports drink can put 30 g of sugar in your system – as much as a chocolate bar. Even coconut water is filled with carbohydrates. If you only get a short workout, a sports drink could actually make you weigh more at the end of a workout than when you start.

Not eating after a workout or eating only protein-rich foods

Many people are particularly afraid to sit down to a proper meal after a workout. Understandably, they don't want all their hard work at the gym to go to waste by eating a meal and putting all those calories back in.

This approach overlooks one little detail – a healthy meal puts more into your body than just calories. It supplies your body with vitamins, minerals, carbohydrates and other nutrients. When you deny yourself a well-balanced meal, you make it difficult for your body to heal itself. In the end, working out and denying yourself a decent meal can lower your metabolism and make injuries a frequent occurrence. You could find it difficult to get regular exercise then. While a good workout doesn't make it okay for you to gorge on anything you want, it does make it okay for you to eat a full meal.

A balanced meal is what you need – not one that arbitrarily stresses on one or another food group. Many people who work out particularly favor proteins. They read that proteins are important to healing the muscles after a workout and go all out on them. Concentrating on proteins to the exclusion of other sources of nutrition, though, can slow down muscle growth, too.

TIP #28: WHY CONSISTENCY MATTERS MOST FOR GETTING FITTER AND HOW TO BE MORE CONSISTENT

It's easy to stick with an exercise program when you first start out; moving your body is new and there's a novelty to lacing up your exercise shoes and launching into a heart-thumping work-out. But how do you feel a few weeks later when the novelty wears off? You might find yourself making excuses not to work out or shortening your sweat sessions. Pretty soon, days go by without working up a sweat and you fall back into old sedentary habits that do nothing for your health or fitness level.

In a world where people expect instant gratification, this situation is all too common. Guys and gals start a fitness program with a bang, and it ends with a whimper--and then nothing. Despite good intentions, it's back to the couch without the incredible benefits that exercise offers.

Why Consistency Matters
Consistency can make all the difference in whether you get fit or stay the same. Next after consistency comes patience. It takes time to see the difference in fitness, not to mention a change in weight and physical appearance.

How can you avoid this fate? Choose a fitness program or activity you can sustain. What's the key to sustainability? Enjoyment and satisfaction! Select something that brings joy, or at least you don't mind doing, and start slowly. You're more likely to stick with it if you start slow, maybe 10 minutes per day, and expand your training from there. Make a goal that's specific, achievable, and sustainable.

Know What You Enjoy and What You Don't

Make sure the exercise you choose suits you and your personality. For example, if you hate to run, running shouldn't be an option, even if your best friend does it and tells you it's the best way to stay in shape. Maybe for her or him it is, but not necessarily for you. Make a list of sports and fitness activities you enjoy and choose from that list.

If you're an outdoor person, think about exercise you can do in nature such as hiking or canoeing. You can even get an effective workout at a local park. Take a brisk walk or jog around the perimeter and then use a park bench to do exercises like push-ups and triceps dips by placing your hands on the bench. Choose an exercise you enjoy, and it will make all the difference in whether you succeed and are consistent.

If you like exercising and socializing, find an exercise buddy to work out with you or join a club focused on some aspect of physical activity. Most areas have hiking, walking, running, and cycling clubs where you can hook up with other people who enjoy the same activity and have similar goals. The extra stimulation of being around like-minded people will motivate you and help you stay consistent.

Vary Your Workouts to Stay Motivated

Another reason people become less consistent and throw in the towel is they get bored. Exercise won't always be pleasant, but it shouldn't bore you. Don't be afraid to vary your chosen fitness routine by trying new workouts. Just be sure you do enough exercise to boost your heart rate in your cardiovascular training zone. Also, make sure you're doing some form of strength training two or three days each week to build strength and preserve muscle mass.

Stay challenged too. On some days, add an extra challenge to your workout. Increase the speed at which you walk or tackle some hills when you walk or cycle. Extra challenge, in moderation, is what helps you get fitter, faster, or stronger and ensures you stay motivated. Remember, motivation is one key to consistency. If you do the same workouts over and over, your body will adapt to that workout and you'll stop making improvements in fitness. Boredom will follow close behind. Your brain and body thrive on trying and accomplishing new things.

The Bottom Line

Are you ready to get started and stay consistent this time? Try these suggestions and make fitness a lifetime habit, rather than something you do for a few weeks and then stop entirely. Exercise offers benefits throughout a lifetime and you'll never enjoy the returns unless you stick with and stay consistent.

TIP #29: FIVE EFFECTIVE
WAYS TO STAY CONSISTENT
WITH YOUR WORKOUTS

So, you've made the big decision to exercise. After years of "planning" on starting an exercise program that never seemed to materialize, you're taking the plunge. Congratulations! It's never too late to get into shape and change your fitness level and life. The benefits of a regular exercise routine are many -- it can help improve both your physical and mental health and even delay the onset of certain age-related illnesses.

The Importance of Exercise Consistency
It's clear that exercise is a powerful prescription for health and well-being but sticking with it isn't always a piece of cake. Even the pros will tell you it's easy to make excuses and get off track, even if you have the best intentions. It takes an ongoing commitment to show up every day to train and move your body consistently.

The good news? There are ways to make exercise consistency a habit. By instilling healthy habits, you'll be more likely to stick with your exercise program in the long-term. While it may not be easy in the beginning, it will become a part of your life if you push through the initial idleness. It's true what they say: The hardest part of exercising is lacing up your exercise shoes. Once you get rolling, momentum helps you keep moving forward.

The key to any goal is consistency. When you are consistent with your training and diet, you are more likely to reach your goals. But how can you maintain that consistency when you have a busy life and other commitments?. Here are some strategies for keeping being consistent with your workouts.

Schedule Your Workouts

Your health is as important as your job, even more so. Without health, you won't be as effective on the job or you might not be able to work. That's why it's important to treat our health with the same respect and concern as your job. Make it a priority! One way to do that is to schedule your workouts, so you're committed to showing up, just as you have to show up at your job. Once it's on your schedule, you won't have excuses when that day rolls around and you have a billion things on your agenda. Also, research shows exercising at the same time each day increases the odds of success.

Know Your Why

Unless you have a compelling reason to get more active, you're unlikely to follow through. Most people have vague, poorly defined reasons they need to exercise, and those reasons aren't convincing enough to get them off the couch. Sit down with a journal or a piece of paper and think about why you need to exercise. Doing it to "be healthy" is too vague. More persuasive might be that you have a mildly elevated blood sugar, and you don't want to develop type 2 diabetes. But take it a step further. How would type 2 diabetes change your life? It might cause other health problems, like cardiovascular disease, and give you less time to enjoy life with your grandchildren. Get specific with what drives you and you'll be more motivated to stick with exercise.

Take on Less

Big fitness goals will smother and intimidate you. You might want to get fit fast but having that as your goal is a recipe for failure. Think in terms of micro-goals, small well-defined goals that encourage you without the intimidation. Achieving micro-goals will help you build confidence and keep moving forward. Invest in a fitness journal and write your mini-goals down. Start with one or two and build from there. Make them specific too. If your bigger goal is to walk 5 miles, 5 days per week, your mini-goal might be to walk around the block. Mini-goals feel less threatening and you're more likely to follow through.

Be Flexible

Can consistency and flexibility coexist? They can! You're more likely to be consistent with your exercise goals if you give yourself freedom of action. Exercise can be more than a structured workout. If you have a day where you're too tired to lift weights or do a more intense workout, do something active that you enjoy, like take a leisurely walk outdoors. Some people, when they encounter an obstacle, give up entirely. Be flexible enough to modify what you do, based on your schedule and how you feel, but do something to continue moving toward your goal.

Just Start

Nothing can replace action and taking the first step. Some people spend weeks and months planning to exercise and never get started. They invest in exercise equipment they never use and join classes they may never attend. Nothing gets accomplished without taking the first step. Don't let a belief that you can't find the time or lack of motivation keep you from getting fit. If you want to get into shape or start a new healthy habit, take action, even if it's only a small step.

The Bottom Line

It's a no-brainer; if you want to achieve a specific goal, you need to put in the work and be consistent with your workouts. Hopefully, these tips for exercise consistency will help you do just that.

PART C: HEALTHY EATING TIPS

In this section, you'll get the knowledge you need to make healthy food choices. Choosing to practice healthy living habits can go a long way toward preventing diseases. Are you in the habit of making terrible food choices?

TIP #30: HOW DIETS
SHOULD REALLY WORK

We are constantly exposed to new and supposedly groundbreaking diets. The majority of these diets are incredibly restrictive and require significant effort to maintain. Many require the purchase of expensive books, subscriptions or supplements. Nearly all of them fail to educate people on how weight is gained, lost or maintained.

The reality is that diet can be incredibly simple. It does not require any branded products. It just requires a basic understanding of our biology, a set of scales and a little time.

Why we need food

When we eat, we consume calories. These calories are simply a measure of energy. The higher the calorie content of a food item, the more energy that is contained within that item.

It is vital that we consume energy because our bodies are constantly using it up. When at rest, we consume energy at our Basal metabolic rate (BMR). Although we're resting, we still need energy to breath, circulate blood around our bodies, grow our cells, digest food and sustain a variety of other processes.

We are, of course, often not at rest. We frequently move around, contracting and relaxing our muscles. This physical activity accounts for a significant amount of energy consumption on top of our BMR.

Surpluses and deficits

Once you've taken all of the above factors into account, each individual has a daily calorie requirement. Each person's BMR varies based on a number of factors including body composition, age, weight and gender. Energy required for physical activity varies significantly based on a person's level of activity.

There are then three possible scenarios:
- You consume fewer calories than your daily calorie requirement (a calorie deficit)

- You consume at or around your daily calorie requirement

- You consume more calories than your daily calorie requirement (a calorie surplus)

These scenarios then determine whether you lose, maintain or gain weight. This is the case because of how our bodies respond to a calorie surplus or deficit.

When you consume more calories than your body requires, the surplus energy isn't wasted. The human race evolved over millions of years spent struggling to find sufficient food to survive. When surpluses of food were discovered, it was vital that the human body stored the excess energy as early humans lacked the technology to keep food fresh. They also had no guarantee that they would continue to find food, meaning they had to store energy to survive frequent stretches of starvation.

One solution that the human body developed was the storing of energy in fat cells. These cells, which have unlimited capacity, can store any food energy that isn't immediately required for the calorie-consuming processes listed above. This is why overeating can lead a person to develop fat on their body.

When you consume fewer calories than your body requires, the deficit must be made up through stored calories. Although the energy stored in our fat cells isn't the only source of stored energy that our bodies can call on, it is one of the options. The energy required is removed from the fat cells, causing them to reduce in size. A calorie deficit is the only diet that you really need.

Keeping things simple

It may come as a surprise that dieting and fat loss can be explained through such a simple process. No special points, no expensive products - just an awareness of the calorie content of the food that you are eating.

The way in which you choose to apply this knowledge should be determined by the urgency of your diet goals. If you're looking to lose weight relatively quickly and consistently, it is entirely possible to track every calorie that you consume and regularly increase or decrease your daily total based on how your weight and body composition are changing.

Regardless of your goals, an increased awareness of how the food you consume directly influences your weight can make a significant difference to your motivation. Remove the jargon and marketing supplied by diet companies, focusing on the simple internal processes that your body is constantly going through. This understanding can provide you with a sense of control and determination that makes sticking with a diet far easier than you might expect.

TIP #31: SEVEN THINGS TO PUT IN HEALTHY SALADS

Done right, a salad can be a fantastic food, both delicious and healthy. But that's the problem; few salads are actually healthy. Most salads are stocked with high-calorie, high-fat ingredients. Frequently included are rich salad dressings, cheese, and sometimes even bacon. When you are creating your own salads, you want to avoid these pitfalls. Here are seven great ingredients that can make a nutritious salad.

Tomatoes

There are a wide variety of different kinds of tomatoes, almost all of which will taste great in a salad. From cherry, to plum, to heirloom, or even to dried tomatoes, you'll have plenty of choice if you opt for some tomatoes in your salad. Tomatoes are very healthy, being extremely high in the powerful antioxidant lycopene. They also contain plenty of vitamins A, C, and K.

Bell peppers

The mild taste of a bell pepper will pair well with almost any other set of salad ingredients. Bell peppers are great for your health, being rich in vitamin C and antioxidants. In addition, colorful foods like bell peppers make for a much more appealing salad. The visual is an underrated element in the enjoyment of food.

Nuts and seeds

A salad doesn't have to be all vegetable. Adding some nuts or seeds will provide wonderful additional flavor. While nuts and seeds are high in calories and fat, they are very good for you in moderation. That's because the fat found in nuts and seeds is healthy, beneficial, unsaturated fat. Some good nuts to put in a salad include almonds, walnuts, and pecans. For seeds, consider sunflower seeds or pumpkin seeds.

Spinach and/or kale

Iceberg lettuce isn't bad for you, but it doesn't hold a candle to spinach and kale. Dark leafy greens like these are some of the healthiest things in the world and a great base vegetable for a salad. These amazing foods are stocked with many kinds of vitamins and minerals and are among the most nutrient dense of all foods. Health experts agree that almost everyone should eat more dark leafy greens.

Fruit

Fruit of almost any kind will be a welcome addition to a salad. The sweetness of fruit will make for a pleasant contrast with the vegetables that predominate in a typical salad. Fortunately, almost all fruits are very healthy. Some of the best fruits to put in a salad include oranges, grapes, pineapple, pear, watermelon, blueberries, and strawberries.

A healthy protein

The big problem with unhealthy salads is often the inclusion of unhealthy proteins like fried chicken. However, it is possible to enjoy a more substantial, yet still healthy salad. The key is to use a nutritious protein such as tuna, grilled chicken, hard-boiled eggs, salmon, or even tofu. A good protein can transform a salad into an entire healthy meal.

A healthy salad dressing

When making a salad, trade the usual rich, creamy salad dressing in for something better for you. Olive oil is a great choice. A nutritious fat like olive oil will help an otherwise bland salad come alive, while still being good for your health. Balsamic vinegar or a light vinaigrette are other solid dressing choices.

Salad should be a healthy food, especially since a super healthy salad can still taste absolutely great. It's just that most salads aren't. Go against the norm by choosing some of the seven wonderful, good-for-you salad ingredients seen above.

TIP #32: FOUR WAYS TO REDUCE YOUR SUGAR INTAKE

Even if you don't consider yourself to be a big "sweets person," there's still a good chance that many of the foods you eat contain "hidden sugars" - also known as carbs (carbohydrates) that can make your blood sugar spike:

•Bread

•Cereal

•Pasta

•Rice

Furthermore, you might be surprised to find out how much sugar there is in things like juice, ketchup, salad dressings, and yogurt.

Therefore, if you are concerned about diabetes or preventing other problems related to high blood sugar, here are four ways that you can reduce your sugar intake.

1. Cut back on sweets
The first step to cutting back on your sugar intake is to cut back on sweet foods and drinks:

•Cake

•Candy

•Donuts

•Ice cream

•Sodas

•Sugary lattes

In addition to spiking your blood sugar levels, these sugary foods and drinks don't really provide you with any nutritional value.

While eating the occasional dessert is fine, you should instead opt for low-sugar treats like berries or dark chocolate.

2. Read the nutritional information on labels
According to the American Heart Association, the average American adult consumes more than 17 teaspoons of added sugar each day - which is more than double the recommended amount. Unfortunately, many of the items found in your pantry likely contain added sugar. Furthermore, you also consume a lot of nutritional sugars from fruits, grains, and vegetables. Therefore, you need to start checking the nutritional labels to see how much sugar you are actually consuming with each snack and meal.

You might need to find low-sugar alternatives to cook with.

3. Increase your fiber intake
In addition to being good for digestive health, fiber can help reduce blood sugar spikes by slowing the amount of time it takes for sugar to get absorbed into your bloodstream. Therefore, a lack of fiber can be very detrimental to your health if you consume lots of sugary foods and drinks.

Here are a few common foods that are high in fiber content:

•Avocados

•Black beans

•Lentils

•Pears

•Raspberries

•Steel-cut oats

4. Eat more foods that are dense in nutrients

When it comes to cutting back on sugar, you don't always need to cut back on calories. Instead, you should focus on eating more nutrient-dense foods that are rich in proteins and healthy fats.

Furthermore, you don't necessarily need to adopt a low-carb diet to cut your sugar intake. You just need to eat "healthy" carbs":

•Beans

•Nuts

•Seeds

•Whole fruits

Since these foods are rich in vitamins and minerals, eating them will make you feel more full - and reduce your cravings for sweets.

In short, cutting your sugar intake starts with eating fewer sweets. Also, don't forget to check nutritional labels to see how much added sugar you are consuming. Eating more fiber can help you avoid blood sugar spikes, as well as improve your overall digestive health. Furthermore, eating foods that are dense in nutrients are more likely to make you feel full - and less likely to make you crave sweets.

TIP #33: REASONS TO TRY INTERMITTENT FASTING

Intermittent fasting is an eating routine that involves alternating periods of eating and fasting. It has recently gained popularity due to promising research, which indicates it can offer a number of health benefits. It has also proven to be an effective weight control strategy for many people. With a relatively simple and flexible implementation, which doesn't involve any special foods, food restrictions, or exercise program, these potential benefits make it a practice worth considering.

There are multiple options when it comes to practicing intermittent fasting, depending on your personal preference and what makes sense for your lifestyle. Some people choose to only eat for a certain number of hours a day; for example 12 hours each of eating and fasting, or 8 hours of eating and 16 hours of fasting (known as the 16:8 or Leangains method). They may eat normal healthy meals for a majority of the week and then fast completely or severely restrict calories for one or two days a week; the 5:2 diet and eat-stop-eat methods fall into this category. Skipping periodic meals or restricting calories every other day are some other possibilities.

One of the main reasons to try intermittent fasting is its potential positive effects on your health. Studies have shown it can improve cardiovascular function by decreasing triglyceride and cholesterol levels, as well as improving your blood pressure and heart rate. Brain function has also been shown to be positively impacted, due to reductions in inflammation, growth of new neurons, and metabolic changes. Oxidative stress, which leads to an increase in free radicals in the body, can also be reduced via intermittent fasting.

In addition to these positive health changes, intermittent fasting can also help protect against negative ones. Insulin resistance, a key contributor to the development of type 2 diabetes, has been shown to decrease. The cardiovascular improvements that often come with intermittent fasting may decrease your probability of developing heart disease. Chances of developing brain disorders such as Alzheimer's disease may also be lowered. Research has shown that intermittent fasting may decrease your likelihood to get cancer by improving metabolism and cell function.

People interested in losing weight may want to try intermittent fasting. By reducing the amount of time you spend eating, you can reduce the number of calories you ingest. Of course, this assumes you continue to eat a healthy diet, and don't overcompensate for the fasting periods by overindulging during the eating periods. Intermittent fasting can also help improve your metabolism, so the calories you do eat are burned off more effectively. Given the number of different ways to practice intermittent fasting, it can be a flexible diet solution that can be tailored to fit your needs.

One final and exciting reason to try intermittent fasting is its potential to increase your lifespan. The general improvements in health associated with fasting outlined above can all contribute to a person's longevity. Research with mice has shown that restricting their time spent eating can greatly improve their lifespan, results which many believe are also possible in people.

Restricting your time and amount of eating may be an adjustment, both physically and mentally. However, the abundant evidence regarding the positive effects of intermittent fasting suggests that it may be worth trying. Given the wide variety of ways you can go about it, with a little fine-tuning, it can easily be incorporated into your lifestyle so that you can start enjoying these benefits.

TIP #34: FOODS YOU SHOULD EAT TO INCREASE ENERGY AND VITALITY

Feeling a loss of energy, concentration, and mental alertness in the early afternoon is common for many people. In part, this is due to the body's natural circadian rhythms. The energy drop may also be the result of the food you consume. Adults, in general, tend to feel a loss of daytime energy as they age. Remedies to combat afternoon fatigue include taking a short power nap, exercising or going for a walk. These options may not be practical in some situations. A better and longer-term solution can be found by including specific foods in your daily diet.

Consuming a candy bar or a sugary drink is not a real solution. You may get a quick energy boost then feel even more tired when the sugar rush wears off. What your body and brain require are foods that are high in fiber and provide a healthy balance of carbohydrates, protein, and fat.

Grains & Nuts
Your body digests whole grains more slowly than other foods. The benefit is greater stability in both blood sugar and energy levels. Oatmeal, an excellent source of fiber and carbs, provides a healthy way to start your day. Oats, in general, work to reduce the risk of heart disease and provide Vitamin B essential for transforming carbs into energy. Replacing white bread with a whole grain option is also a wise choice.

Brown rice contains a high level of manganese, which breaks down proteins and carbs and converts them into energy. Unlike starchy white rice, brown rice is less processed and contains higher nutritional value. The fiber content helps to regulate blood sugar levels and sustain an even energy level throughout the day.

Walnuts, almonds, and pistachios will all provide a quick boost to your energy level. They contain magnesium and vitamins B and E, which reduce stress and fatigue. Pistachios are high in both fiber and protein. Even peanut butter, when used in moderation, is an energy booster. Choose an all-natural brand to reduce sugar content.

Fruits and Vegetables
Eating one orange not only provides the recommended daily dose of vitamin C but also contributes natural sugars and fiber to sustain energy levels. Oranges contain antioxidants, which can reduce feelings of stress. To obtain the full benefit, you need to consume the entire orange except for the peel. Apples are also a great source for carbs, fiber, and antioxidants. The best results come from eating the whole apple, peel and all, rather than simply consuming apple juice. Bananas offer another energy stimulating option. They provide potassium and electrolytes with the added benefit of high fiber content.

Other energy-producing fruits include raspberries, cherries, blackberries, pears, and strawberries. Fruit works great as a stand-alone snack you can toss in your bag or briefcase or as an ingredient in a salad, on cereal or when combined in a smoothie. Yogurt, which is, by itself, an excellent energy-producing snack containing carbs, protein and important vitamins, can also be enhanced by topping it with your favorite fruit.

If your diet preference tends toward the vegetarian side of the menu, you can choose from a wide selection of items rich in manganese, vitamins, iron, and other energy-producing nutrients. These include asparagus, broccoli, mushrooms, carrots, cabbage, spinach, kale, sweet potatoes, and artichokes.

Fish
Salmon and tuna are often referred to as brain foods. They contain healthy omega-3 fatty acids that have been shown to improve memory, mood, and energy. A tuna sandwich on whole-grain bread provides an excellent energy boost to work through the afternoon. Adding tuna or salmon to a lunch salad also serves to enhance alertness and eliminate feelings of fatigue.

Honey, Chocolate, and Coffee
Consuming a moderate amount of honey will boost your energy in just minutes. Honey contains important nutrients, vitamins, and minerals plus natural sugars. Combine it with oatmeal for a double dose of energy.

Dark chocolate contains a natural stimulant similar to caffeine. Snacking on a small amount can generate a large energy boost plus an improved mood. Antioxidants improve blood flow, which, in turn, increases oxygen to the brain-stimulating alertness and focus.

Coffee is a natural go-to drink for many who feel the need for a little energy boost. The caffeine content, which quickly passes from the bloodstream to the brain, often results in a quick jump in both alertness and focus. An average cup of coffee contains few calories as long as you don't start adding, sugar, cream, and flavorings.

Both the quantity and quality of food eaten during the day impact energy levels. Replacing some of the foods in your diet with these energizing options should result in sustained vitality plus improved concentration and focus, enhancing your productivity all day long.

TIP #35: FIVE POWER FOODS TO GET YOU THROUGH YOUR WORK DAY

Everyone gets hit hard by the afternoon slump. Usually, by 2 p.m., people's heads start to sag just a little at their desks. It's only a few more hours until quitting time, and you can't take a nap unless your company allows it. You need a little pick-me-up. Don't reach for another cup of coffee. The energy from the caffeine won't last. Do not reach for an energy drink, either. Those things can kill you - literally. Power foods are not only healthy for you, they will also pick you up enough to make it to five o'clock. Here are five of them from which you can choose.

Nuts and Seeds

One of the best power foods out there is nuts. Nuts are packed with protein and some varieties add a nice dose of healthy fat to your diet. The best nuts to snack on are almonds and walnuts. Almonds will stabilize your blood sugar and give you consistent energy throughout the rest of the afternoon. Walnuts are a fantastic choice for omega-3 fatty acids, which will boost your brainpower. If seeds are your preference, stick with a healthier option such as pumpkin seeds. These traditional Halloween treats can be eaten year round and they pack a nice punch of magnesium to your daily diet.

Dried Fruit

Something to add to your nuts or seeds is a few pieces of dried fruit. Fresh fruit is also a great option, but sometimes the workplace might not accommodate such a treat. Dried fruit is easy to store - it doesn't need refrigeration - and pops into your mouth without the added stickiness of, say, a juicy orange. Dried apricots are the perfect choice when it comes to this popular dried treat. Apricots boost your glucose safely and naturally, and they also give your body a little extra oxygen-boosting iron. Grab a handful of almonds and dried apricots together. It makes a healthy mini-trail mix and you can dry the fruit yourself.

Hard-Boiled Egg

Eggs got a lot of bad press for a long time, but new studies show the cholesterol concerns initially surrounding the consumption of eggs just might be unfounded. No, you shouldn't eat a three-egg omelet for breakfast every morning and then top it off with a hard-boiled egg in the afternoon, but if you've stuck to a whole-grain cereal for your morning meal, there's nothing wrong with an egg for your afternoon pick-me-up. As long as you can keep the egg in refrigeration until you are ready to eat it, this snack is a healthy power food packed with enough protein to tie both your energy and appetite over until dinner.

Plain Low-Fat Yogurt

Plain yogurt is the only way to go when it comes to yogurt. You'll be surprised to learn that upwards of 1/4 cup of sugar is added to fruit-flavored yogurts. That's right. Fruit-flavored yogurts are absolutely packed with unhealthy sugar, which is not only bad because too much sugar is harmful you, but it also defeats the point of a power food pick-me-up, as you'll crash - hard - after the sugar wears off. The sugar-free yogurts are laden with artificial sweeteners, which have their own health concerns. So, grab a plain low-fat or non-fat yogurt, both excellent sources of protein, and add some frozen cherries or blueberries to make it more palatable.

Edamame

Soybeans are super good for you, and they're also a power food that is perfect for your afternoon snack. Edamame already husked is easy to find at the store; you can even purchase dry-roasted soybeans for a nuttier-type snack. Packed within these little green beans that look a cross between lima beans and peas is a hefty amount of iron and folate, both proven to increase brain function and cognitive performance. Soy also has other health benefits, such as lowering your cholesterol and reducing your risk of heart disease.

If none of these power foods sound appealing to you, keep a few things in mind when looking for your perfect afternoon snack. Select snacks that are high in protein and low in fat; fat makes you sleepy. Avoid foods with unhealthy carbohydrates, such as sugar-laden foods. Make sure your snack isn't too big. If you load up on calories in the afternoon, even healthy ones, you'll still need that nap. And finally, do snack. Our bodies work much more efficiently when they are fueled throughout the day, so keep your metabolism running with some healthy power snacks.

TIP #36: TEN BEST WAYS
TO EAT FRUIT

With its sweet, succulent flavors, fruit is one of the most popular foods around. It's also one of the most healthful. But many people don't get the full benefits of eating fruit simply because they're unaware of the best way to do it. Whether you're a daily fruit consumer or an occasional indulger, these ten tips will help show you how to eat fruit to gain all the advantages it has to offer. You won't just enjoy the experience more; you'll give your body a noticeable health boost too.

Choose High-Nutrient Fruits
Fruit comes in all shapes, sizes, colors, and nutrient levels. If you want to get the most nourishment from eating fruit, go for the varieties packed with vitamins, minerals, and antioxidants. Berries top the list, thanks to their plentiful polyphenol antioxidants, vitamin C, fiber, and manganese. Other notable powerhouses include kiwi, pomegranates, grapefruit, apples, and oranges. Best advice? Eat an array of fruits to ensure you get a range of nutrients.

Go Organic, Especially for These
There's been much debate about whether eating organic food is worth the cost. When it comes to fruit, you'll avoid harmful pesticides by choosing organic varieties, but studies suggest you might also consume higher levels of nutrients. For some people, organic fruit is worth the price based on taste alone. A good rule of thumb is to go organic for the fruits listed in the Environmental Working Group's Dirty Dozen: strawberries, apples, peaches, pears, nectarines, cherries, and grapes.

Wait for Fruit to Ripen

There's more reason than better flavor to wait for fruit to ripen. Scientists believe that doing so increases the antioxidant levels present in the fruit. Be wary of letting fruit ripen too long, though. Those brown bananas sitting in your fruit bowl may be perfect for banana bread or muffins, but they've also undergone nutrient loss that makes them less valuable for health. One benefit of eating underripe fruit is that it may contain more fiber than its more mature counterpart.

Clean Your Fruit First

Washing produce before eating it helps prevent food-borne illnesses, which is why the Center for Disease Control recommends cleaning your fruit prior to consumption. But this simple habit can also remove residue, dirt, and other debris that gets stuck on fruit and makes it taste bad. What about fruit with peels or skin you don't plan to eat? They still need a good rinse for cleanliness. The best way to clean fruit is to wash it under running water and dry it with a paper towel or cloth.

Chop It Up

Grabbing an apple or banana on the run might seem like the simplest and most convenient way to eat fruit, but taking the time to chop it up and sit down to enjoy it can make a big difference to your taste buds and health. You'll help improve the digestive process that way, plus it's less messy, more filling, and easier to avoid damaged or bruised areas. You'll also appreciate the aroma, flavor, and texture of fruit better when you chew leisurely and pay attention to your senses.

Don't Overeat Fruit

According to the USDA, adults should eat at least five servings of fruit daily. While that may sound like a lot, a serving size isn't all that big--roughly 80 grams, the size of a small orange or a half-cup of chopped fresh fruit. In fact, it's easy to consume more than five servings in a day. There's no harm in doing so as long as you avoid consuming large quantities of fruit, which can cause stomach upset and keep you from getting nutrients from other important food groups.

Be Wary of Juices

Fruit juice can count for a daily serving of fruit, but it's not always the best way to consume fruit. Many fruit juices contain added sugar and preservatives that make it less healthful than whole fruit. Plus, you miss out on the fiber benefit of eating a piece of fruit. Of course, every fruit juice is different, and some contain ideal nutrition. Read labels before choosing fruit juices. Or, do your own juicing to get all the benefits of whole fruit without the harmful additives.

Consider Frozen Fruit

Picked right off the crop or purchased from your local farmer's market are great ways to get the freshest fruit, but don't discount the frozen section of your grocery store. Many frozen fruits are picked at their peak and frozen immediately to retain nutrients in their richest condition. Frozen can be the ideal way to get summer fruits during the wintertime, too. When fresh fruit doesn't look so fresh, head to the freezer. You may be surprised at the varieties and quality you'll find there.

Eat Fruit Between Meals

Diet experts agree that eating fruit between meals is a healthy habit worth following. That's because fruit is a filling snack that satisfies and keeps hunger pains at bay. Eating fruit on an empty stomach can also help process the nutrients better than eating fruit during meals. Some people swear by starting the day with a piece of fruit and a glass of water as the best way to give your body an energy boost. No matter when you time it, eating fruit daily will give you health perks.

Get Creative

Fruit is highly versatile, which makes it a fun ingredient for your culinary dishes. Cooking, baking, and grilling with fruit is all the rage today. Try fruit skewers on the barbecue, make a healthy fruit crisp for dessert, or mix fruit into your favorite casserole or salad. There are many ways to get creative with fruit and boost the nutritional profile of your meals. Look online for recipes, then get busy creating healthy fruit concoctions for you and your family to enjoy.

Eating fruit regularly is an excellent health habit, but to make it even better, follow the above tips. The rewards will be that much sweeter.

TIP #37: THE TRUTH ABOUT SUGAR IN FRUITS - WHY FRUIT SHOULD FORM A PART OF EVERYONE'S DIET

The first step for many people when trying to eat a healthier diet is to eat less sugar. There is a proven link between high sugar consumption and problems ranging from obesity to dental health. Many people's first thought would be to cut down on soft drinks and sugary treats, but there is also a worrying trend suggesting that people should avoid fruit due to its high sugar content.

Why Excess Sugar is Bad

Excessive sugar intake is known to cause a whole range of problems, one of the most damaging being obesity. Obese people show an increase in instances of heart disease, type 2 diabetes, digestive issues, and some forms of cancer. In some countries, it has reached such a level that a sugar tax is present to reduce the harmful impact.

The problem mainly lies with added sugar, the type found in soft drinks, and sugary treats. Products with a large quantity of added sugar have little to no nutritional benefit and do not cause a feeling of fullness. This lack of fulness means that people keep on drinking or eating other foods, and consume far too many calories.

Why Sugars in Fruit Are Different

Almost all fruits contain a large amount of sugar. Not only this but the sugar in fruits, known as fructose, has the same effect on your body as the sucrose that makes up table sugar. However, the difference is in the context. Fruit contains other nutrients and minerals, and so is not nutritionally worthless.

Importantly, fruit contains a lot of fiber. Your body cannot digest fiber, and so the fruit is broken down steadily in the stomach, causing a slow release of sugar, and a feeling of fullness. This satiety stops overeating, and dramatically reduces the risk of obesity.

Can You Have Too Much Fruit?
It is almost impossible to eat enough fruit to cause problems relating to the sugar content. The amount needed to introduce issues is way above the recommended level, and you would need to eat almost nothing else! As part of a balanced diet, the sugar levels in fruit are of no risk to the majority of the population.

What About Tinned or Processed Fruit?
The one exception is where the fruit is processed and packaged with added sugar, such as syrup. This sort of preservation destroys a lot of the nutritional value of the fruit, although the fiber content remains roughly the same. That said, tinned fruit is undoubtedly better for you than a can of soda!

Dried fruits such as raisins also get a bad reputation, even though they have virtually the same nutritional profile as the grapes from which they came. As part of a balanced diet, they are an excellent source of many nutrients. The problem lies in controlling the portion size. Dried fruit takes up a fraction of the volume of the hydrated fruit, making it very easy to overeat.

There is no reason to be worried about the sugar content of fruit, as long as you balance your diet by eating plenty of other food types. You can gain the most benefit by varying the types you eat to give you as much nutrient diversity as you can. Like every part of your diet, the key is moderation and variety. If you stick to that principle, then anything you like to eat can form part of your diet.

TIP #38: NUTRITION FOR BEAUTY: 9 ESSENTIAL NUTRIENTS FOR SKIN, HAIR, AND NAIL HEALTH

No matter your age, nutrition affects your appearance in many ways. If you don't get the essential nutrients your body needs, your hair, skin, and nails will suffer. Eating plenty of natural, highly nutritious foods will ensure you get everything you need for a radiant appearance. Below is a list of beauty nutrients that can help you eat your way to a glowing, more youthful version of yourself.

1. Vitamin A
Vitamin A renews and repairs cells, membranes, and tissues. It's great for reducing wrinkles and maintaining smooth, glowing skin. It also controls the activity of the sebaceous (oil) glands to promote scalp health. Other benefits include protection against UV skin damage and preventing collagen breakdown. If you don't get enough vitamin A, your skin may appear dry, itchy, and bumpy. Excellent food sources for this nutrient include sweet potatoes, carrots, pumpkin, spinach, collard greens, cantaloupe, and squash.

2. Vitamin B Complex
Several B vitamins have substantial beauty benefits; B3 encourages ceramide and fatty acid production, compounds that make up the skin's protective barrier. It is also essential for DNA repair. B5 moisturizes and nourishes the skin, and strengthens hair follicles. B6 protects the skin from dryness, and it gives your hair a vibrant color. B7 (biotin) increases nail thickness and protects

hair by preventing thinning and split-ends. Finally, B9 (folate) assists in cell repair and DNA synthesis. You can find an abundant of B vitamins in lentils, cereals, eggs, red meat, chicken, fish, broccoli, and asparagus.

3. Vitamin C

Nature's incredible antioxidant defender protects against free radicals that cause dark spots, sagging, and wrinkles. Vitamin C is also vital for collagen and elastin production; these substances keep the skin toned and firm. It protects from sun damage and makes your complexion brighter while it renews damaged skin and treats pigmentation. This essential nutrient also replenishes vitamin E in the body. Foods rich in vitamin C are bell peppers, papaya, broccoli, Brussels sprouts, strawberries, kiwifruit, oranges, and pineapple.

4. Vitamin D

Another nutrient that assists in skin regeneration is vitamin D. It prevents dryness and promotes softness while making the skin more robust and less susceptible to sagging and wrinkles. Vitamin D also plays a role in controlling the natural antimicrobial defenses of the skin. There are broader benefits as well as it enhances immunity and improves mood. You can find vitamin D in dairy, tuna, soy milk, orange juice, and by making sure you get some sunlight during winter.

5. Vitamin E

As an antioxidant and anti-inflammatory compound, vitamin E protects against free radical damage. It also absorbs UV light energy and defends against skin cancer. It works well with vitamin C to promote cell integrity. All in all, vitamin E is essential for moisturized skin and a healthy scalp. Some foods rich in this beauty nutrient are almonds, avocados, chard, olives and olive oil, peaches, spinach, tomatoes, and sunflower seeds.

6. Omega-3 Essential Fats

Essential fatty acids are natural anti-inflammatory agents and very helpful for several conditions, such as acne, psoriasis, rosacea, and wrinkles. Omega-3s keep your skin firm, moist, and flexible. They also inhibit the activity of a specific chemical that encourages the spreading of skin cancer. They prevent hair and scalp dryness and protect against collagen loss. Make sure you eat enough oily fish, such as salmon or sardines, walnuts, flax seeds, tuna, wild rice, and edamame.

7. Potassium

Potassium is an essential mineral that maintains pH balance in the body. It supports healthy circulation, muscle and nerve function, and it promotes new cell growth healing blemishes and scars. It's also one of the nutrients that smooth out wrinkles and protect from UV rays. Some foods high in potassium are beans, bananas, salmon, avocados, yogurt, and chard.

8. Selenium

Selenium is a superb free-radical fighter that preserves skin elasticity and protects against skin damage. Moreover, selenium deficiency has been linked to a higher risk of skin cancer. Brazil nuts are by far the best food source of this mineral, but you can also find it in decent amounts in oats, mushrooms, tuna, shrimp, salmon, and wheat germ.

9. Zinc

Zinc is a mineral that plays a crucial role in collagen formation and tissue healing. It combats inflammation and redness and assists in sebum production, promoting healthy hair and nails. It also protects against conditions like acne. It's a mineral found in high concentration in the outer layer of your skin. As an antioxidant defender and potent skin healer, zinc can slow down the aging process and protect your skin from free radical damage. You can find zinc in oysters, red meat and poultry, dairy, mushrooms, chia seeds, chickpeas, pumpkin seeds, tahini, quinoa, and hemp seeds.

Essential vitamins and minerals provide countless beauty benefits for skin, hair, and nails. They are nature's way of helping you always look your best. Furthermore, essential nutrients promote optimal health, protect against disease, and boost your energy levels. Eating a variety of nutrient-dense foods will help you stay healthy, energetic, and radiant. So, if you are looking for the fountain of youth, look no further from your plate.

TIP #39: TEN EASY WAYS TO GET MORE BENEFITS FROM THE VEGETABLES YOU EAT

Non-starchy vegetables are powerful sources of antioxidants and dietary fiber. These are components that help your body maintain a healthy immune system, balance blood sugar levels, and regulate bowel movements. Eating non-starchy vegetables will also provide more vitamins and minerals than you can get from most other foods.

Unfortunately, most people don't eat enough of them, and you might not be getting the full health benefits from the ones you eat. Need some guidance? Here are 10 simple ways to get more health benefits from the vegetables you eat.

Eat Some Raw Vegetables to Maximize Vitamin C
There are benefits to eating both raw and cooked vegetables, but you'll get more vitamin C from those that you eat raw. Vitamin C is sensitive to heat or light, and if you cook vegetables, particularly in large amounts of water and at high temperatures, you'll lose 40% or more of their vitamin C content.

For example, broccoli is an excellent source of vitamin C. However, studies show that vitamin C levels when you cook it. For instance, boiling broccoli lead to a 54.6% drop in its vitamin C content, while steaming lowered vitamin C by only 14%.

You also lose some B-vitamins when you cook vegetables for a long time, or expose them to high heat. However, cooking can also make some nutrients, such as beta-carotene and lycopene, more bioavailable. So, eat both cooked and raw veggies. For example, a study found that heating tomatoes boosted their lycopene content by 35%.

Choose Colorful Carbohydrates

If you have a choice between a starchy carbohydrate and a colorful vegetable, choose the latter. Color is a marker of a healthy array of phytonutrients that have benefits that go beyond simple nutrition. Some have antioxidant and anti-inflammatory activity that you won't get from their less colorful counterparts. So think color! Colorful vegetables are often easier on your blood sugar too. For example, potatoes cause a sharper rise in blood glucose than eating a colorful veggie like red cabbage.

Add a Source of Fat to Your Vegetables

Fat isn't the enemy. In fact, adding modest quantities of healthy fat to a veggie plate or salad has benefits. For example, you'll absorb more beta-carotene, a precursor to vitamin A from a salad, if you include a healthy source of fat. Cold-pressed olive oil, avocado, cold-water fish and flaxseed are good sources of healthy fats. Avoid processed vegetable and seed oils, like soybean oil, corn oil, and sunflower oil.

Make Your Veggies Easy to Prepare

Food processors make chopping vegetables easier, so keep one on the counter for faster prep. Add your veggie ingredients to the food processor, and pulse until chopped into smaller pieces. This is a great way to enjoy vegetables without doing too much work! When it's less work to prepare them, you're more likely to eat them.

Buy Frozen Vegetables if You Can't Eat Them Quickly

If you buy fresh vegetables and can't eat them before they spoil, consider buying frozen ones. Frozen vegetables are harvested at their peak, providing the nutrients of fresh vegetables with added convenience. Freezing prevents further nutrient loss, so the nutrients are preserved even if you keep them in the freezer for weeks. In contrast, fresh vegetables sit on store shelves and lose nutrients, such as vitamin C.

Substitute Noodles for Veggie Noodles

Vegetable noodles are nutrient-dense replacements for regular pasta. Switch white noodles for ones made of vegetables like zucchini, sweet potato, and yellow squash that are fabulous better sources of nutrients and easier on your blood sugar. Replace white rice with cauliflower rice for more vitamins, minerals, fiber, and antioxidants. It's an easy step you can take to easily meet your veggie quota.

Grow Your Veggies in a Container Garden

Grow your own vegetables in a simple container garden. You can grow quite a collection of veggies if you have a small balcony or patio. Try growing spinach, lettuce, kale, tomatoes, watermelon, peppers and herbs. With such easy access, it'll be easy to get your veggie quota each day. You don't need a plot of land to grow vegetables, a patio with sunlight is enough to grow many vegetables.

Make a Veggie-Based Smoothie

Start the morning with a low-sugar smoothie, but include a handful of greens, such as spinach or kale. You won't notice the taste of the leafy greens, as the fruit will mask it. Add a small amount of ground flax seed to your smoothie. It will provide you with essential fatty acids, as well as lignans, which offer powerful anti-cancer properties.

Eat Veggies As Soon As You Wake Up in the Morning

The earlier in the day you start eating your veggies, the more likely you are to get your five plus servings. Why not start with breakfast? Switch that bagel for an omelet loaded with veggies. You'll get hunger-satisfying protein combined with veggies such as mushrooms, bell peppers, broccoli, spinach, and any other colorful veggie you can include.

Add Vegetables to Other Foods

Upgrade the veggie content of mashed potatoes by replacing half the potato with pureed cauliflower. Add pumpkin to your bowl of oatmeal in the morning and to pancake mix for more nutrition, and an extra serving of fruit and veggies. Change your side dishes too. Skip the starchy side of rice or potatoes and replace it with a colorful vegetable. Easier on your blood sugar and waistline too!

The Bottom Line

Hopefully, these tips will help you get more vegetables on your plate and into your body. Enjoy the added health benefits you'll get by eating more plant-based foods.

TIP #40: SIX WAYS TO A HEALTHY IMMUNE SYSTEM

The human body is remarkable in its ability to fight off the many viruses, germs and diseases that strike it on a daily basis. A healthy immune system works day and night to eliminate foreign invaders. However, factors such as a high stressed lifestyle, poor diet and lack of exercise interfere with the body's ability to function, leaving it vulnerable to disease. Even worse, the extensive use of prescription and non prescription drugs adds to the overload of chemicals already in the body. A detox program and the use of natural herbs and the elimination of toxins helps to boost the immune system,

Echinacea

It's been known for its ability to fight colds and the flu far better than any vaccine or drug can accomplish. While the medical community insists that everyone take flu shots, too often the vaccine fails to provide any protection and often brings about severe side effects. Because we pump our bodies with chemicals such as thimerosal that contains 50% mercury, we only weaken the immune system.

Ginger

In use for thousands of years in China, ginger was the solution to digestive disorders. Ginger is a simple herb that is used as a tea and flavor meals. It's a better alternative to antacids that only suppress stomach acids. While antacids help subdue heartburn and indigestion, they destroy the beneficial flora that keep Candida overgrowth and bad micro flora from flourishing in the stomach.

Garlic

It's a "super food" that has been studied and tested extensively. It helps boost the immune system as it is one of nature's most potent antibiotics. Its anti-bacterial and anti-viral qualities are well known, yet this herb is seldom found on the average American plate. No drug ever devised can boast the added benefits of reducing cholesterol and improved circulation.

Healthy Teas

Green, white and black teas have many health benefits including improved immune functioning. They contain high levels of antioxidants, even more than many vegetables.

Elimination of Refined Sugars

The elimination of refined sugar in the diet is one of the best ways to restore a healthy body and mind. Unfortunately, most of today's foods come loaded with sugar, fats and other chemicals that wreck havoc on the digestive and immune systems. Sugar has been known to kill many of the beneficial bacterial flora in the intestines. Without a healthy gut, good health is impossible. A constant diet of refined carbohydrates leads to diabetes and heart disease.

Regular Exercise

Regular activity improves circulation and helps eliminate the toxins that accumulate in the body's fat tissue. A healthy immune system depends on an active flow of blood to every part of the body that carries the oxygen needed by all the organs to function. Regular exercise helps reduce colds and prevents the onset of the flu.

These six simple methods can help restore an effective immune system. They can help cut down on the use of standard medications that too often mask but never eliminate disease.

TIP #41: COULD A VEGAN DIET GIVE YOUR IMMUNE SYSTEM A BOOST?

Your immune system works hard to protect you from all sorts of deadly diseases. So, anything that can give your immune system a boost is something that you need to know about. A vegan diet could actually make your immune system stronger. To find out more, keep reading.

- **Food Matters:** Your diet impacts your health. One way of figuring out how your diet impacts your immune system is to understand that your immune system is your body's main system of defense against disease. For example, if you consume food that regularly adds carcinogens into the diet, your immune system needs to work overtime to neutralize the effects of these unhealthy substances and prevent these substances from causing cancer. Now, working overtime regularly reduces productivity among workers. So, it stands to reason that a diet which is full of unhealthy substances makes the immune system work overtime. This is likely to lead to an immune system that is not as productive as it could be. Now, unhealthy diets were linked in a research study to the deaths of 400,000 people who died from heart disease. The researchers who conducted the study recommended adding a heap of whole grains, veggies, seeds, and nuts into diets to prevent similar deaths. All these foods happen to be totally vegan.

- **Plant Powered Wellness:** People who opt for a plant-based diet seem to fall ill less frequently than those who follow meat-based diets. Lots of research studies have identified that vegetarians and vegans do have stronger immune systems when compared to people with meat-based diets.

- **Live Longer:** Vegans tend to live longer than non-vegans, according to a study that monitored 131,342 people for more than 25 years. Increased plant protein in the diet was linked with a significant reduction in the risk of death. The consumption of red meat has been found to increase the risk of death due to a variety of diseases in several comprehensive studies. However, there is insufficient research on the impact that dairy foods can have on health and longevity, and some studies indicate that certain types of dairy could promote health.

- **Skip the Carcinogens:** Non-vegan diets have been found to contain many unhealthy substances that have been linked to diseases that are usually fatal. For example, both the consumption of red meat and the consumption of processed meat have been found to add carcinogens, which are chemicals that increase the risk of cancer, into the diet. Carcinogens are created when meat is cooked and when meat is processed. Vegan foods do not contain substances that have been linked to chronic diseases such as heart disease and cancer. This is why the consumption of certain types of vegan food is usually recommended as a means to reduce the risk of deadly diseases such as heart disease and cancer.

It seems that plant powered foods are linked with stronger immune systems, longer lives, and cleaner diets. Yet while a vegan diet can have an incredibly positive impact on your health, all non-vegan foods are not made equal. Among non-vegan foods, certain types of dairy have been shown to have a positive impact on health. But opting for a vegan diet can surely give your immune system, which does the heavy lifting in protecting you from deadly diseases, a big boost in the short term.

TIP #42: SEVEN SIMPLE WAYS
TO ADD MORE HEALING
FOODS TO YOUR DIET

Healing foods are nutrient-dense food choices that contain additional phytonutrients, compounds that have antioxidant and anti-inflammatory activity. There's some evidence that eating more of these foods may protect against chronic health conditions related to aging, such as cardiovascular disease and type 2 diabetes, as well as slow the aging process itself. One theory as to why aging occurs is cell and tissue damage due to oxidative stress.

It's easiest to add more healing foods to your diet by making small changes. The purpose of this chapter is to show you simple ways to replace some of the foods you currently eat that are low in nutrient density with ones that are more nutrient-dense. Let's look at some super-simple ways to add more healing foods to your diet.

Add Produce to Your Morning Meal
The earlier in the day you start eating nutrient-dense fruits and vegetables, the more likely you are to get your five-plus servings of fruits and vegetables in. If you eat a bowl of oatmeal or whole grains cereal, add your favorite berries and a pinch of cinnamon to help with blood sugar control. Rather than serving eggs, make a veggie omelet packed with vegetables such as mushrooms, tomatoes, spinach, garlic, onions, red peppers, and more. With eggs and veggies, you get fiber and protein for satiety but also vitamins, minerals, and antioxidants.

Have a Smoothie "Snack"

Some smoothies have a bad reputation as being too high in sugar, but if you make one at home with the right ingredients, it doesn't have to be. Unlike juice, you retain the fiber when you make a smoothie. The key to making a smoothie that won't spike your blood sugar is to choose a high ratio of vegetables to fruit. For example, make a smoothie with spinach, kale, and blueberries. Although it will have a green shade, the berries will mask the taste of the greens. If you want it a little sweeter, add a natural calorie-free sweetener like Stevia. Frozen berries work well for making green smoothies and you can combine them with your favorite plant-based milk.

Watch What You Drink

Get the most out of the beverages you sip too. The worst thing you can drink is soft drinks and other sugar-sweetened beverages. You're probably aware that drinking too many sugary beverages can lead to health problems, such as obesity and dental cavities. But should sugary drinks be avoided altogether? The answer, in most cases, is yes. The American Heart Association recommends limiting added sugar to no more than half of your daily discretionary calorie allowance.

Why not make your go-to beverage green tea? Some research suggests that green tea has healing properties, thanks to powerful antioxidants called catechins, which help prevent cell damage. Studies are looking at whether the antioxidant power of green tea could lower the risk of some health problems, like cardiovascular disease, cancer, or dementia. The verdict is still out but sipping a cup of green tea is a smarter option than drinking a beverage high in sugar.

Replace the Starch and Double Up on the Vegetables

Starchy foods, like white rice, white potatoes, and pasta are favorite side dishes for many people, but these foods are low in nutrition relative to colorful, non-starchy fruits and veggies.

There's an ongoing debate in the nutrition community about the potential health benefits and/or risks of starchy foods, like white rice, white potatoes, and pasta. While these foods are a good source of energy, they can also be high in calories and carbohydrates.

You can up the nutrient content of any meal by replacing these starchy options with a colorful vegetable. If you like the taste of white rice, try cauliflower rice, available frozen at many grocery stores. It has the same look and texture of rice, but it's made from diced cauliflower, a more nutrient-dense option. How about spiralized zucchini in place of pasta noodles? If you cant give up baked potatoes, switch that white potato for a sweet potato or a purple sweet potato. You'll get more nutrients per bite.

Upgrade Your Salads

Start each meal with a salad. Studies show that doing this can reduce the number of calories you eat with the rest of your meal. Swap the iceberg lettuce for more nutrient-dense healing foods such as kale, watercress, and cabbage. Add artichokes, carrots, red peppers, and mushrooms for more nutrients and healing power. Top it off with a sprinkle of broccoli sprouts, one of the richest sources of glucosinolates that your body converts to anti-cancer compounds.

Add More Spices

Did you know gram for gram, spices have more antioxidant power than fruits and vegetables? When you speak of healing foods, it would be inconsiderate not to mention herbs and spices. Many, such as rosemary, garlic, turmeric, cinnamon, and oregano, have antioxidant and anti-inflammatory activity. There are many different types of spices and each one offers a different set of health benefits. Your best bet might be to eat a variety. If you're on blood thinners, talk to your doctor before using some spices, such as garlic, since it can interfere with the benefits of these medications.

Eat Local

Eating "local" may means something different to each person. For some, eating locally may mean sourcing your produce from directly from a local farm. For others, it may mean purchasing locally grown produce at the supermarket. Either way, the common theme is that the food is grown or produced close to home. If you eat local, you know that fresh local food tastes better. But did you also know that eating local helps you eat healthier? Eating local food is good for your health because it's more nutritious.

Why is locally grown food more nutrient-dense? When food travels a shorter distance, there's less time for it to lose its nutrients. Some vitamins are especially sensitive to heat and light, such as vitamin C and some B-vitamins. So buy close to home and use your produce as quickly as possible.

The Bottom Line

Use these simple ways to add more healing foods to your diet to upgrade the nutrient density of what you eat. Healing foods are satisfying and delicious!

TIP #43: IS SODIUM BAD FOR YOUR HEALTH? THE SALTY TRUTH ABOUT SODIUM AND HOW IT AFFECTS THE BODY

Millions of Americans follow a low-sodium diet, believing it will protect them from heart disease, kidney disease or osteoporosis. While sodium consumption can play a role in these and other chronic ailments, it's still an essential nutrient the human body needs to function properly. If you restrict your body from sodium, it can have a rippling effect on your health.

Sodium vs. Salt: What's the Difference?
The terms "sodium" and "salt" are often used interchangeably, but they aren't the same. Sodium is a mineral with the atomic number 11 that all people and animals -- as well as some plants -- need to function properly. Salt, on the other hand, is a mineral consisting of roughly 60 percent chloride and 40 percent sodium. There are different types of salt, including table salt, sea salt, Himalayan salt and kosher salt, but there's only a single type of sodium.

Why Sodium Is Essential for a Healthy Diet
As an electrolyte, sodium protects against involuntary muscle contractions or spasms by providing your body with electrical energy in the form of charged molecules. The nervous system tells muscles when to contract and relax using electrical signals. If you have a sodium deficiency, the lack of charged molecules will affect how your nervous system communicates with your

muscles, which could lead to spasms.

When consumed, sodium is quickly absorbed into the bloodstream to protect against low blood pressure. It increases your blood volume, which causes the pressure inside your veins to rise. People who struggle with hypotension are often advised by doctors to consume more sodium in their diet to help raise their blood pressure.

Adequate sodium intake also protects against a potentially serious medical condition known as hyponatremia. Defined as a low ratio of sodium to blood, it's a leading cause of emergency room visits in the United States. With hyponatremia, fluid inside the bloodstream moves to nearby cells, including brain cells, where they cause cells to swell.

Symptoms of hyponatremia include:
- Headache
- Fatigue
- Lethargy
- Nausea
- Lightheadedness
- Muscle cramps or spasms
- Memory loss
- Confusion
- Seizure
- Coma

How Excessive Sodium Intake Can Adversely Affect Your Health

Although it's essential to your health, sodium can have adverse effects when consumed in excess, such as high blood pressure. The kidneys can filter sodium from the blood. But if you overburden your kidneys by consuming too much sodium, the mineral will accumulate inside your bloodstream where it causes your blood pressure levels to rise, thus increasing your risk of hypertension-related ailments like heart disease and stroke.

Because the kidneys are responsible for filtering sodium from the bloodstream, a high-sodium diet can increase your risk of kidney disease. The kidneys work by pulling unwanted fluid from the blood via osmosis and channeling it to the bladder. For this to happen, your body needs a proper balance of sodium and potassium. Consuming too much sodium or too little potassium restricts your kidneys' ability to pull unwanted fluid. And high blood pressure caused by the over-consumption of sodium will compress your kidneys and their blood vessels, further increasing your risk of kidney disease.

Consuming too much sodium can increase your risk of the chronic bone disease osteoporosis by filtering an excess amount of calcium from your blood. Calcium is the primary mineral used in the production of new bone tissue. When sodium levels in your bloodstream are high, your kidneys will pull both sodium and calcium to discard as waste. And without a plentiful of calcium, your body will then pull this mineral from your bones, resulting in a loss of bone density.

High-sodium diets have also been linked to digestive problems. Because of its antibacterial properties, sodium is used as a preservative in many packaged foods. Sodium still retains its antibacterial properties when consumed, meaning it kills the colonies of good bacteria in your gut. As your gut flora is affected, bad bacteria can thrive unchecked to cause digestive problems like constipation, bloating and diarrhea.

How to Moderate Your Sodium Intake
Statistics show the average person consumes about 3,400 mg of sodium per day. In the 2015 to 2020 Dietary Guidelines for Americans, however, the U.S. Department of Health and Human Services (HHS) recommends consuming just 2,300 mg per day. To avoid its potentially harmful effects, you must moderate your

sodium intake by staying within this daily limit.

Limit your use of salt when preparing and cooking food. One teaspoon of table salt contains up to 2,325 mg of sodium, which is already more than the daily intake recommended by the HHS. To satisfy your taste buds without consuming an excessive amount of sodium, consider using a salt substitute. It has a similar taste, but contains other minerals, such as potassium chloride, instead of sodium.

Whether you are shopping for groceries or dining out at a restaurant, be proactive toward identifying the sodium content in the foods you eat and the beverages you drink. In the United States, chain restaurants are required by law to display the nutrition information, including sodium content, of the foods and beverages they sell.

There are six foods, specifically, that contain extremely high concentrations of sodium. Dubbed the "salty six" by the American Heart Association (AHA), they consist of breads, pizza, soup, deli meat, poultry and tacos or burritos.

Condiments like ketchup, mustard, barbecue and soy sauce can pack a significant amount of sodium. One tablespoon of ketchup, for example, contains 154 mg of sodium, while one tablespoon of soy sauce packs up to 879 mg of sodium.

Increasing your potassium intake can help counter the effects of sodium. Potassium stimulates your kidneys, causing them to flush more sodium from your blood. Along with cutting back on salt, choosing high-potassium foods can curb the effects of high sodium consumption.

Sodium isn't a junk ingredient that's used strictly to improve the flavor or shelf life of foods and beverages. It's an essential nutrient that protects against muscle spasms, low blood pressure, osteoporosis, digestive problems and hyponatremia, all while balancing your body's fluid levels. By moderating your intake of sodium, you'll reap these health benefits without experiencing its harmful effects.

TIP #44: CONGRATULATIONS ON YOUR LOW SALT DIET

Your doctor has just told you to go on a low salt diet, or technically, a low sodium diet. Perhaps you have high blood pressure. Perhaps you have Meniere's disease. Whatever the reason, you have been warned that you have to cut down on your consumption of sodium.

There's no question that suddenly reducing salt from your diet will cause some inconveniences, especially if you are around others who still want to eat salt. Your family may complain. Going to restaurants becomes difficult, as does eating with friends.

All of these facts may seem like reasons to be depressed, as you contemplate giving up pretzels for what may be the rest of your life. However, a low salt diet has many positive sides. In fact, even if a medical professional has not ordered you to reduce the salt in your diet, you may want to consider doing it anyway. Here are some benefits to reducing your sodium intake:

You will feel less bloated.
Your body usually tries to maintain a certain level of sodium in your bloodstream. When you consume excessive sodium, your body compensates by retaining extra water. As you cut back on sodium, your body will not hold onto as much water. Depending on where you start, you will probably lose a pound or more as your body releases the water.

You may lose a little weight, especially at first.
If you're accustomed to eating salty food, suddenly switching to

food with little or no salt will be disappointing for your taste buds. Therefore, you will probably consume less food and a few pounds will melt away. Another reason for losing weight will be the fact that salty snacks, such as popcorn or potato chips, are addictive; once you start eating, it can be difficult to stop. However, if you never take that first handful of potato chips, you don't have to worry about taking a second.

You're going to eat less processed food.

Most dietary sodium comes from processed food, such as bread, pizza, cold cuts, bacon, potato chips, many kinds of cheese, and cookies. You also have to be careful of canned goods and raw chicken, as both can have salt added to them. In other words, you're going to have to read the labels (or check online, when the labels are too small). However, the easiest approach to consume less sodium is to consume food that is natural and unprocessed, such as eggs, dairy, vegetables, and fruit. Why is eating less processed food beneficial? Because processed foods are usually not just overloaded with salt, but with many other chemicals that may be bad for you. You may be avoiding sodium in order to lower your blood pressure, but the change in eating habits may help you avoid cancer, too.

Your taste buds will adjust.

At first, the reduction in salt will taste weird, but most people's taste buds do adjust. The food with too much salt for you will taste as if it has too much salt. This is a good sign. It will help you avoid the foods you should avoid, and you will no longer feel as if reducing your sodium intake is a burden. Always look at the label; however, some processed foods contain sodium without tasting salty.

You're going to discover some great flavors.

Instead of eradicating the taste of everything with salt, you will give your taste buds the chance to appreciate more delicate flavors. Squeeze lemons or limes on your food, or experiment with various low sodium spices. For example, you can put cinnamon instead of salt on popcorn to make it interesting. To get you started, here are the milligrams of sodium per tablespoon for various spices. Basil has 0 mg, cinnamon has 1 mg, garlic has 6 mg, and turmeric has 10 mg. Alas, some spices will still have to be avoided, such as onion salt or any other seasoned salt. Chili powder has 131 mg of sodium per tablespoon, while soy sauce contains a whopping 879 mg. However, after your taste buds adjust, you won't want the high sodium spices anyway.

On average, Americans consume 3400 mg of sodium per day, while the daily recommended allowance is only 2300 mg. Note this is the recommendation for someone who weighs 150 pounds. If you weigh less, you should consume even less sodium, or your doctor may have recommended a lower limit. By restricting your sodium, you will be healthier, and your new eating habits may inspire a healthier approach to salt in your family and friends, too.

TIP #45: FIVE EASY WAYS TO EAT MORE PROTEIN WITHOUT SUPPLEMENTS OR POWDERS

Protein is an important macronutrient that builds and maintains muscle, helps you feel full, and provides your body with key vitamins and nutrients. Protein is also generally leaner and more filling than other food sources, which helps stabilize blood sugar and insulin and helps lead to fat loss.

However, it can be difficult to get enough protein in your diet, especially since contemporary Western diets are often dominated by low-quality foods high in processed carbohydrates, sugars, and greasy fats. Depending on your size or activity levels, you should try to eat between 80 to 180 grams of protein daily.

Try these five easy ways to consume more protein without resorting to powders, shakes, or supplements.

1. Eat the Meats
It is no secret that meat is one of the best sources of protein possible. Here is approximately how much protein you can find in 100 grams or 3.5 ounces of the following meats:
- Chicken and Turkey: 30 grams
- Beef: 26 grams
- Lamb: 25 grams
- Pork: 27 grams
- Sardines: 25 grams
- Tuna and Cod: 23 grams
- Salmon: 20 grams

3.5 ounces is just a little less than a quarter pound and is roughly the same size as a smartphone. Rather than eating a lot of meat in one sitting, try eating a moderate amount at each meal or cutting it up and adding it to sandwiches or salads. Try to get meats that are organic, non-processed, non-GMO, grass-fed, or wild-caught (for fish) to get the best possible quality.

2. Get Egg-Cited

Eggs are lean, tasty, quick to prepare, and are an excellent low-calorie source of protein. An average egg will contain about 6 total grams of protein - approximately 4 grams of protein in the white and 2 grams of protein in the yolk. Larger or jumbo sized eggs will have up to 8 grams of protein per egg. Try to get local pastured or organic eggs for the best quality.

Eggs are easy to make and are an excellent choice for any meal, especially breakfast or lunch. Eating eggs in the morning can help you start off the day with a filling and satisfying meal and just 4 eggs can provide 24 to 30 grams of protein. Adding eggs to salads or as sides to meals can also be a convenient and delicious way to increase your protein consumption.

3. Go Nuts

Nuts are easy to eat and are high in protein and can be an excellent option for healthy snacking. Pretzels, chips, and crackers are filled with processed carbohydrates, sodium, and empty calories. Nuts are just as crunchy and delicious and provide your body with far better nutrients.

Replace your junk snacks with nuts to simultaneously cut down on empty calories while also consuming more protein. If possible, purchase non-GMO or organic. The following popular nuts have some of the highest amounts of protein per ounce:
- Peanuts: 7 grams
- Almonds, Pistachios: 6 grams
- Cashews: 5 grams

- Walnuts, Hazelnuts, Brazil Nuts, Pine Nuts: 4 grams
- Pecans: 3 grams
- Macadamia: 2 grams

4. Dabble in Dairy

Even if you're lactose intolerant or prefer to avoid dairy, you may want to try some high-protein dairy options. One cup of milk has 8 grams of protein, but more solid and fermented dairy products such as cheeses or yogurts contain even more. These products also contain less lactose as much of it is lost or drained away during processing. Many of these products are available organic, non-GMO, or with limited amounts of antibiotics or hormones. Here are the protein contents of several healthy dairy and cheese options:

- Kefir: 11 grams / cup
- Yogurt: 12 grams / cup
- Greek Yogurt: 22 grams / cup
- Parmesan: 10 grams / ounce
- Romano: 9 grams / ounce
- Low-Fat Swiss or Low-Fat Cheddar: 7.5 grams / ounce
- Nonfat Mozzarella: 7 grams / ounce
- Provolone or Gouda: 7 grams / ounce

5. Help Yourself to Whole Grains

Despite recent low-carb crazes, eating moderate amounts of non-processed, complex whole grain carbohydrates is healthy and necessary. Whether it's bread, pasta, or side dishes, eat these protein-packed whole grains instead of the common nutrient-poor white or processed variety. Many whole grains (with the exception of wheat) are also naturally gluten-free. Here is the protein content per cooked cup of some popular whole grains:

- Quinoa: 8 grams
- Whole Wheat Pasta: 7 grams
- Wild Rice: 6.5 grams
- Millet: 6 grams
- Oatmeal: 6 grams

- Buckwheat: 6 grams

Regardless of your goal, increasing the protein in your diet can help you feel healthier, stronger, leaner, and better nourished. By adding some of these healthy protein sources to each meal or snack you can increase the quantity of your overall protein intake without purchasing shakes, powders, or supplements.

TIP #46: FIVE WHOLE GRAINS THAT ARE GOOD FOR YOU

You've probably heard that you should eat whole grains rather than foods made from processed white flour, but do you know why eating this way is good for you?

It's because whole grain is food in its natural state where the seed is kept whole rather than ground up. There are three parts of the seed that is edible, the endosperm, the germ, and the bran.

Each of these parts holds essential nutrients unlike processed grains such as white bread, white pasta and white rice that have been milled to take away the germ and bran and leave only the endosperm.

The reason this is done is that it gives the product a finer texture and a longer shelf life. In the process, it also takes away its essential nutrients. So, whole grains should always be your choice and you can find them in many different forms including cereals, flour, pasta, rice, and bread.

What nutrients do they contain?

Because eating whole grains is so beneficial to your health, most nutritionists recommend that you eat three servings daily. But even if you only eat one serving a day, it has been shown that you will have reduced your disease risk. Whole grains are essential for weight management because of the high amounts of fiber that they contain. This fiber helps regulate your blood sugar and will make you feel fuller longer. In addition, whole grains are full of minerals such as iron, selenium, and magnesium and B vitamins such as folate, thiamin, niacin, and riboflavin.

Do whole grains help prevent disease?

Yes, this is absolutely true. The Whole Grains Council has stated that eating whole grains can reduce your chances of heart disease by 25-28 percent, Type 2 diabetes by 21-30 percent and stroke by 30-36 percent. These are huge numbers and need to be taken seriously.

Which grains are the healthiest?

1. Quinoa

Quinoa is not only healthy but it tastes very good. It is different from other grains in that when it's cooked it becomes fluffy and light and it cooks quickly compared to other grains. Also, its flavor is not overwhelming so it can be combined with other foods. Quinoa is high in protein and low in fat. It also helps regulate cholesterol levels, aids digestion and can help fight off some types of cancer. In addition, it is a great energy source and helps reinforce and strengthen glands, organs, and muscles.

2. Brown rice

As an alternative to white rice, brown rice is the healthy choice. It is more nutritious because it is unprocessed. It is also protein-rich and contains B vitamins and fiber. With its essential nutrients that are not found in many other foods, it is an excellent supplement to your diet. For example, gallstones can be prevented by the fiber that brown rice contains and it is recommended for anyone who might be developing gallstones.

3. Whole oats

If you are trying to add more calories to your diet, whole oats are an excellent choice. That's because 1 cup of whole oats has over 600 calories. Whole oats are also rich in fiber. In fact, one cup will provide 67 percent of the recommended daily fiber intake for adults. They also contain high amounts of iron and protein. When you eat whole oats for breakfast you will feel full longer and they will help keep you from eating again before lunch. Whole oats are also a great source of energy and cooked whole oats help to regulate blood sugar. So, they are good to help prevent type 2 diabetes, cardiovascular disease, and obesity.

4. Barley

Another excellent grain source is barley which has a nutty, hearty flavor that complements almost any food and it has a consistency similar to pasta. One of the advantages of eating barley is that it is low in calories and full of essential nutrients such as manganese, selenium, phosphorus, iron, copper, protein, and fiber. The biggest drawback to eating barley is that it takes a long time to cook so it isn't as convenient. But, if you plan ahead and set aside the time it takes to cook, it's worth the trouble. That's because it also reduces the fat known as visceral fat which surrounds your vital organs. As a result, barley is highly recommended if you are trying to lose belly fat.

5. Millet

Another very healthy whole grain is millet. This is a very small grain that comes in many colors including gray, red, yellow or white. It also has a good, delicious taste and can be eaten mashed or whole. As with many other whole grains, millet is high in nutrients such as fiber, phosphorus, manganese, and protein while being low in calories. Its magnesium content makes it helpful in maintaining heart health.

Finally, it helps reinforce and develop body tissues and lowers the risk of type 2 diabetes. So it is an important food for pre-diabetics and people who are prone to developing gallstones.

Conclusion

For all of these reasons, try whole grains because chances are you will love them. And best of all, they don't have the low carb problems like their alternative, white grains.

TIP #47: WATER OR ELECTROLYTE DRINKS: WHICH IS BETTER FOR THE BODY?

Electrolyte drinks are all around us, and as consumers we are constantly bombarded by their advertisements on television and elsewhere. Their advertisements claim to restore the energy lost during tough workouts and to help athletes perform better. One of the most common electrolytic drinks is Gatorade, which is bought by millions of people throughout the world. But many wonder whether or not these drinks claim to do the miracles of restoring energy that they claim to do. Is it really worth it to buy these drinks when it is much cheaper to just drink water?

The truth about sports drinks greatly depends on the amount of physical activity that you do on a daily basis. This is because electrolyte filled drinks are filled with mainly two ingredients. These are carbohydrates and of course electrolytes. Carbohydrates make up many of the Calories that we consume on a daily basis because just one gram of carbohydrates make 4 Calories. If you are not someone who works out on a daily basis, consuming the extra Calories is unnecessary and for that reason alone, sports drinks should not be in your diet.

Sports drinks are also filled with electrolytes. When advertised on television, electrolytes seem to be something that should be in every one's diet. However, this is not necessarily the case. Electrolytes are essentially salt, and more specifically, they're sodium. The average person in the U.S. consumes way too much salt and sodium on a daily basis and they should not be taking in any more than they already are. The average sports drink has over two-times the amount of sodium than what is found in an average glass of soda. This excess sodium is not needed for athletes who are trying to perform at their best.

Even though there are multiple down sides to drinking sports drinks, there are a few instances when they can be helpful. Mainly after a workout has just been completed, it is very important to consume a lot of carbohydrates. Consuming carbohydrates is very important after a workout because after a workout there is a one hour time period in which newly consumed carbohydrates can transform into any nutrient that your body may need. A good goal to aim for after a workout is consuming 60 grams of carbohydrates. This is where sports drinks come in. If you drink a sports drink within an hour after you finish a workout, then the large amounts of carbohydrates in that drink can be turned into any nutrient that your body may need. Sports drinks are not the only source to get the carbohydrates that you need because many foods are filled with carbohydrates. This means that sports drinks do not have to be the only source for your carbohydrates and they are not necessary to drink as an athlete, but they can be drank if the time is right.

The best choice for athletes and other people who exercise is water. Water has zero Calories and no carbohydrates or sodium. Overall, water will hydrate you just as well as any sports drink on the market while helping you to avoid the downsides. Another upside to drinking water is that it is much cheaper than sports drinks when you buy a filter from the store and filter your own water at your own home.

Overall the best option for an athletic drink is water. Sports drinks can be nice after a workout, but they are unnecessary and can be costly. If you want to perform at your best, you should drink water over any other type of sports drink in order to save you money and perform at your best.

TIP #48: THE KETO DIET: DOES IT REALLY WORK FOR WEIGHT LOSS?

Are you trying to lose weight? If so, you might be wondering whether the keto diet will help. Characterized by a low intake of carbohydrates, it's become one of the most popular weight loss diets in recent years. With the keto diet, you'll essentially replace carbohydrates with fat. While the thought of consuming more fat may sound counterproductive, this isn't the case. The keto diet can, in fact, help you lose weight by transforming your body's metabolism.

What Is the Keto Diet?
The ketogenic diet, or what's more commonly known as the keto diet, is a low-carbohydrate, high-fat diet that's designed to stimulate the human body's natural fat-burning mechanism. Under the keto diet, most of the calories you'll consume will come from fat. You can still consume protein as well, but the keto diet embraces a low intake of carbohydrates and a high intake of fat.

The keto diet was pioneered by the Mayo Clinic's Dr. Russel Wilder in the 1920s as an alternative treatment for epilepsy. Wilder found that epilepsy patients experienced fewer seizures after replacing a large portion of carbohydrates in their diet with fat. In the years to follow, medical researchers discovered other benefits of the keto diet, including weight loss.

How the Keto Diet Can Help You Lose Weight
The keto diet receives its namesake from the metabolic state it induces: ketosis. After following a strict keto diet for about two to six days, your body will enter ketosis in which it pulls energy

from stored fat. As your body continues to burn its stored fat, you'll lose weight. The keto diet leverages the fat-burning mechanics of ketosis to promote weight loss.

The human body demands energy to function properly. Whether you are mowing the lawn, working in the office or even sleeping, your body needs energy. The keto diet encourages your body to use stored fat for energy rather than glucose.

According to the U.S. Centers for Disease Control and Prevention (CDC), Americans get about half of their daily calories from carbohydrates on average. Carbohydrates, of course, are processed into glucose by the liver. When you consume them, your liver will produce and release glucose, resulting in elevated blood glucose levels. In response, your pancreas will produce and release insulin to help your body use and store the excess glucose. If your insulin levels are high -- a common problem with high-carbohydrate diets -- your body will store glucose as fat.

The keto diet promotes weight loss by lowering your blood insulin levels. When you restrict your body of carbohydrates, your body will pull energy from glucose stored in the liver and muscles. Once those reserves are depleted, your blood insulin levels will drop while forcing your body to pull energy from stored fat instead.

Is the Keto Diet Safe?
While effective at burning fat, the keto diet does pose some safety concerns. Since carbohydrates are the main source of fiber for most Americans, for instance, you may experience digestive problems. Constipation is a common side effect reported by individuals on the keto diet. With a low intake of carbohydrates, you may consume an insufficient amount of fiber, resulting in constipation or other digestive problems.

You may experience mental and physical fatigue while on the keto diet. As you restrict your body of its normal source of energy, you may feel more exhausted than usual. This mental and physical fatigue, however, is short-lived and typically subsides after a few weeks.

Ketoacidosis is another concern associated with the keto diet. It's a more extreme form of ketosis in which ketone levels rise to dangerous levels. While on the keto diet, your liver will break down stored fat into ketones, which are then used as energy instead of glucose. Because they are acidic, ketones will alter the pH level of your blood. As ketones build up, your blood will become dangerously acidic to the point where it causes nausea, stomach pain, vomiting, dehydrating or even coma.

With that said, the keto diet shouldn't result in ketoacidosis if you follow it correctly. Your liver will still produce ketones, but it won't produce an excessive amount of ketones that could otherwise lower your blood's pH to a dangerous level.

Keto Diet Tips for Success
To lose weight with the keto diet, you must selectively choose foods and beverages that are low in carbohydrates and high in fat. When most think of carbohydrates, they envision bread, pasta, rice and potatoes. But carbohydrates come in many forms, including simple sugars. Soda, for instance, often contains over 30 grams of carbohydrates, all of which come from sugar, whereas bananas contain 27 grams of carbohydrates. For your body to enter ketosis in which it burns stored fat, you must avoid all high-carbohydrate foods and beverages.

There are plenty of keto-friendly foods that you can eat. Cheese is an excellent keto-friendly snack that's low in carbohydrates and high in fat. Depending on the variety, it may contain some sugar in the form of lactose, but it's not enough to raise your body's glucose levels high enough to trigger weight gain. Cheddar, gouda, mozzarella, parmesan and swiss are some of the best varieties for the keto diet because of their low lactose content and, therefore, low carbohydrates.

Along with cheese, other keto-friendly foods include:
- Eggs
- Nuts
- Leafy greens
- Flax seeds
- Pumpkin seeds
- Sesame seeds
- Blackberries
- Blueberries
- Mushrooms
- Raspberries
- Avocados
- Beef
- Chicken
- Turkey
- Pork
- Fish
- Shrimp
- Lobster
- Crab
- Olive oil
- Coconut oil

Whether artificially or naturally sweetened, you shouldn't drink sugary beverages while on the keto diet. Instead, drink either water or a non-sweetened beverage, such as tea or coffee.

Keto isn't the only low-carbohydrate diet. Others include the Atkin's and paleo diets. The keto diet is distinguished from its counterparts, however, by an exceptionally low intake of carbohydrates. You may get up to half of your daily calories from carbohydrates while on the Atkin's or paleo diet, compared to just 10 percent while on the keto diet. By slashing your intake of carbohydrates, you'll force your body to burn stored fat for energy.

TIP #49: COULD A LOW CARB LIFESTYLE BE THE BEST WAY TO ACHIEVE YOUR WEIGHT LOSS RESOLUTION?

At its peak of popularity in the early 2000's, the low carb diet was seen as something of a bizarre fad. Due to the number of celebrities rumoured to be following plans like the Atkins diet, and the way it was often portrayed in the media that low carb dieters lived off of cheese, bacon and little else, many were doubtful about whether this style of diet had any scientific reason for working, and were concerned about its long term health effects.

Now the celebrity low carb trend seems to have passed, it is a good time to re- evaluate this diet objectively. In truth, low carb dieting has been practiced for over 50 years, and is based on strong scientific principles. If you have tried more mainstream 'low calorie' or 'low fat' diets with little or no success, then low carb may well present the means for you to finally meet your weight loss goals, and it is also ideal for bodybuilders who want to cut fat and show off their muscles. However, you do have to truly understand how low carb dieting works, and follow it rigidly to ensure it works as planned and does not compromise your well being.

Why Do Low Carb Diets Work?
The human body is designed to be able to run on two different sources of fuel. The fuel it chooses first is glucose. Glucose comes into the body when you eat carbohydrates, and is stored in your muscles as a substance called glycogen, ready to be used when you move. The secondary source of fuel the human body can run

on is fat, which, unsurprisingly, enters your body when you eat fat, and is stored in your body as fat. The body runs just as well on either of these fuels, though due to the nature of glucose, when you are powered by this you may experience peaks and troughs in energy relating to when and what you eat, caused by blood sugar 'spikes'. You don't get these when your body is running on its fat supply.

If you want to lose some of the excess fat in your body, then, the most efficient way to burn it off is to switch your body from being a glucose burning engine, to a fat burning one. The only way to do this is to deprive the body of carbs, and allow the glycogen stored in your muscles to be used up to nothing (a process which for most people takes two or three days). Once your body has begun to burn fat, it will continue to do so as long as there isn't enough glucose coming in to tip the balance back. Burning fat leads to rapid weight loss.

What Do Low Carb Dieters Really Eat?
On a low carb diet, eating fat is not only not seen as a bad thing, it is crucial, because that is what your body is running on (and even if you have plenty of fat available in your body, you will go into 'starvation mode' if you aren't eating one fuel source or the other, and this will hamper your weight loss). Low carb dieters therefore get to eat some things that people on a conventional diet would refuse. They are advised to leave the skin on chicken when they eat it. They can, in most cases, eat cheese (some low carb dieters find cheese delays weight loss, but most can tolerate it). They can eat fatty meats like pork, duck and lamb without concern. The high fat content may make the low carb diet look unhealthy to outsiders, but remember that these are mainly natural, whole foods, not that different to what our ancestors who hadn't worked out how to mill flour and make bread yet would have eaten.

Even in the very restricted, early stages of a low carb diet, the dieter can have some carbs (on Atkins, for example, you can have 20g a day of carbohydrate in the two week induction phase). This is not very much, but smart low carb dieters know to maximise the benefits they get from their carb allowance by using it to accompany their proteins and fats with leafy green vegetables. Eating greens keeps their fiber levels up, helps feed them with vitamins, and makes their meals feel more complete.

Is Low Carb Suitable For You?
Low carb living is something just about anyone can do, as after a little research, it is easy to remember and follow the rules. However, there are some people it tends not to suit so well, because it doesn't meet their energy or taste needs. People who work out a lot may find that a standard, low carb diet doesn't give them the fast burning energy they need to get their best performance, and may be better advised to try an adapted version like the Targeted Ketogenic Diet where you only eat carbs before heavy activity. People who have a very sweet tooth may find the diet hard to stick to, because there are only limited sweet foods you can have (even fruit is high in carbs). Vegetarians and vegans may also struggle to have an interesting and fulfilling low carb diet, because so many low carb recipes are based around animal proteins and fats, but it is not impossible.

If you want to start seeing the benefits of the low carb way of life for yourself, then the best place to start is to read up as much as you can about the science behind it and how to implement it in your life. Then, set a date and get started!

TIP #50: FARMERS MARKETS:
A FRESH IDEA

If you have been out and about lately, you have probably noticed a wonderful trend-- farmers markets are popping up all over the place. Like scattered sunflower seeds, farmers markets are sprouting here and there, bringing delight to every neighborhood where they appear. Farmers markets are fun, outdoorsy places where you can gather all the fresh produce you need for the week. Depending on your location, you will find scrumptious seasonal veggies, from artichokes to zucchini. If you live within driving distance of an orchard, grove or berry farm, you will find an assortment of delicious fruit at your nearby farmers market. Quite often, local bakeries peddle their fragrant wares alongside vendors of olives, herbs and freshly cut flowers.

There are several good reasons to shop at neighborhood farmers markets. Obtaining your fruits, flowers and vegetables directly from the people that grow them supports your local economy. Why purchase from big grocery chains and support big, out-of-state corporate farms when you can buy local goodies grown with love?

When you visit a local farmer's booth, you can learn about what goes into growing their fruits and veggies and many growers offer tasty recipes, as well. At the Carlsbad, California farmers market, there is a woman who grows sweet basil hydroponically and sells it wrapped in newspaper like an old-fashioned flower bouquet. Her handmade hempseed and pine nut pesto is the best, so if you see her at a southern California farmers market, be sure to give her perfect pesto a try.

Of course, buying fresh-from-the-field vegetables is a good enough reason to patronize your local farmers market, but a morning or afternoon spent strolling the stalls is a fun social event, as well. Something about being outdoors, surrounded by booth after booth of delicious fresh produce, seems to bring out the best in people. Everyone from energetic kids to little old ladies enjoys the fresh air and camaraderie of a farmers market. Many patrons of farmers markets are regular visitors, and soon you may be, too. Get to know your local farmers and you're bound to make some new friends.

If you are a vegan or just appreciate plant-based meals, you can plan your week's menu around the treats that you find at your neighborhood farmers market. Everyone knows that veggies are good for you, but big corporate grocers sell a lot of genetically modified produce, so you can never be sure what you're buying. Virtually all farmers market vendors grow organically and the difference is remarkable.

Wear your best straw hat, grab a canvas shopping bag, slip into some comfortable shoes and have a delightful day exploring booth after delicious booth. Get some sunshine and tasty things to eat at the same time. Farmers markets are a fresh idea whose time has come.

TIP #51: TWELVE INGREDIENTS THAT ARE KILLING YOU – AND YOU DON'T EVEN KNOW IT!

By now, anybody with access to basic media knows that too much of just about any food can be bad for your health. What fewer people know is that for some foods, any amount could be too much. The problem is that Americans get their food recommendations from the Department of Agriculture – a government agency tasked to increase the profits of American agribusinesses. This is different from increasing the health and lifespan of the American population. Would you like to guess who loses when those two points come into conflict?

That's right. You lose. Especially if your food contains one of these twelve secretly deadly ingredients.

1. **Propyl Gallate** is intended to protect you from eating rancid oils and fats. It acts as a preservative, extending the shelf life of foods like vegetable oil, soup stock, breakfast cereal, candy, chewing gum and potato snacks. Some people are allergic to propyl gallate, meaning it may exacerbate asthma or even cause anaphylactic shock like you see with peanut allergies. In the long term, studies demonstrate a link between propyl gallate and stomach irritation, liver damage and kidney problems. Some research also shows a link to increased chances of cancer.

2. **Hydrogenated Vegetable Oil** is an object lesson in unintended consequences. Back when people thought all fats were bad and all cholesterol was deadly, hydrogenated oils like margarine were thought to protect people from heart disease. Since

the 1990s, though, nutrition science understands that hydrogenated oils – also called trans fats – are worse for you than the saturated fats found in butter and red meat. They directly contribute to your risk for heart and circulatory problems like stroke, high blood pressure and heart attack.

3. **Diacetyl** may seem familiar to you after reports in 2007 that it sickened workers at a food processing plant, killing many of them outright. Since then, many food manufacturers have announced removing this butter substitute from products like microwave popcorn. This is good news, right? Seems like it, until you realize that those manufacturers have replaced diacetyl with "diacetyl trimmer" which releases diacetyl in the presence of heat and water – in other words, whenever you cook it.

4. **Olestra** provides the flavors and consistency to food that you normally get with fat. It has zero calories, and your body is incapable of absorbing it. Knowing that, it should come as no surprise that it's become a staple ingredient in diet snacks. However, olestra can cause digestive problems ranging from irritable bowels to nausea to painful cramping. Worse, it blocks your body's absorption of beta-carotene, lycopene and lutein. Since these nutrients are instrumental in protecting you from killers like cancer and heart disease, olestra does more than upset your tummy.

5. **Aspartame** is an artificial sweetener you'll find in diet sodas, low-calorie ice cream and similar diet sweets. It's part of a long line of artificial sweeteners that turned out to be dangerous – after millions had consumed snacks containing the chemical. Aspartame can trigger migraines, hallucinations and neurological dysfunction. Long-term exposure has been linked to greater risk of cancer.

6. **High Fructose Corn Syrup** is a subtle poison, a sugar that's present in more processed foods than you're likely to imagine.

It not only increases the caloric content of a food, but it blocks your ability to realize you're hungry. That's right – it means more calories in food, and eating more of that food. With obesity-related disorders making up 3 of the top 5 killers in America, and a growing diabetes epidemic, this food may just turn out to be the deadliest thing on supermarket shelves this century.

7. **BHA & BHT,** also know as butylated hydroxyanisole, is another additive used to preserve fats in foods. You'll find it in foods like beer, breakfast cereal, butter, chewing gum, dehydrated potatoes, gum, meats, potato chips and vegetable oil. It's been linked to cancer in lab studies on rats, with human testing just around the corner.

8. **Potassium Bromate** improves the action of flour during food processing – making it less expensive to make processed foods that include flour. Science has known this food additive promotes cancer of the kidney and thyroid for twenty years. It's illegal in many countries because of this obvious health hazard. The United States is not one of those countries.

9. **Sodium Nitrite/Nitrate** sees use in the meat packing industry. It's an additive that improves color and enhances flavor, most common in preserved meats like bacon, sausage and ham. Sodium nitrite/nitrate is like that one kid you knew in high school. It doesn't cause cancer on its own, but it encourages compounds to form during cooking – and those compounds do cause cancer. It can also encourage the growth of botulism, a deadly food toxin responsible for hundreds of deaths every year.

10. **Saccharin** is one of the original artificial sweeteners, used in diet sodas and low-fat snack foods. It has been conclusively linked with cancer of the ovaries, urinary tract and bladder. Its deadly reputation has taken it off the list for high-profile foods like most diet sodas in America. However, you'll still see it in off-brands in the United States, and used frequently abroad.

11. **Food Coloring** isn't always deadly, although you can make the argument that it's never necessary. The bad news is that it's almost impossible to find foods without food coloring. The good news is that only a few are actually poisonous. Blues #1 and 2, Red #3 and Yellow #6 have been shown to cause cancer, and to increase the cancer-causing properties of other carcinogenic compounds.

12. **BPA, or bisphenol A,** is not a food. It's a powder used in numerous plastic products including your reusable food containers and baby bottles. Studies link BPA to increased risk of breast cancer, dysfunction in the brain, heart and thyroid, obesity, infertility, diabetes and several forms of cancer. You can identify containers with BPA by the number 7 in the recycling triangle.

The best defense against deadly food is to cook from scratch using simple ingredients your great-great-great grandmother would recognize as food. Barring that, it's essential to read food labels at the supermarket. If you find these ingredients, put an item back on the shelf.

TIP #52: WHY EATING A MEDITERRANEAN DIET IS A TIME-TESTED STRATEGY FOR BETTER HEALTH

It's one of the most diverse diets in the world with an abundance of whole foods. The Mediterranean diet offers a wide variety of tantalizing and flavorful foods and compelling health benefits too. In fact, many populations of the world who live to a ripe old age eat a traditional Mediterranean diet. A number of studies link eating a Mediterranean-style diet with a reduced risk of heart disease and stroke. That, in and of itself, is a strong reason to eat a traditional Mediterranean diet.

What is the Mediterranean Diet?
The Mediterranean diet emphasizes fruits, vegetables, nuts, seeds, legumes, and fish. Olive oil is not just used for frying and for dipping bread. It is used to cook and flavor a variety of Mediterranean offerings. This style of eating may, based on correlational studies, lower the risk of heart disease, stroke, and obesity.

There are many ways to eat a Mediterranean-style diet. Some recipes are more elaborate, though they don't require a lot of expensive ingredients. For example, a day might start with scrambled eggs and tomato sauce, or with yogurt with berries and honey. A simple recipe for lunch or dinner is vegetables grilled in olive oil. The dishes typically look as appetizing as they taste as well. The emphasis is on unprocessed foods that are low in sugar. Fish is the preferred protein source, with lesser amounts of poultry and little red meat.

The Mediterranean Diet is Nutrient Dense and Fights Inflammation

Obesity is another risk factor for cardiovascular disease. Being extremely overweight is unhealthy to the heart in many ways. Plus, carrying too much body fat increases the risk of type 2 diabetes, hypertension, and lipid abnormalities. Why is excess fat problematic? It produces chemicals that boost blood vessel-damaging inflammation. Some studies show that the Mediterranean diet reduces inflammation, and it's a delicious way to do it.

For example, a study of 600 adults over the age of 65 found those who ate a Mediterranean diet experienced a drop in markers of inflammation as well as beneficial changes to the composition of their gut microbiome. Researchers say these changes may lower the risk of insulin resistance, fatty liver, and certain types of cancer. Once the participants stopped eating the Mediterranean diet, their gut microbiome returned to its former state.

Also, the Mediterranean diet is a rich source of fiber, vitamins, minerals, and healthy fats, all of which are associated with helping to protect against obesity as well as the conditions that contribute to it. The Mediterranean diet is different from the more common Western diet in that it tends to be plant-based. Plant foods are high in dietary fiber, help to maintain a healthy gut, help to produce hormones that control hunger, and keep blood sugar levels down. Whole grains and legumes are very high in fiber. This can help to reduce the risk of heart disease and type 2 diabetes.

Specific to the Mediterranean diet is the health-promoting vitamins and minerals found in the abundant variety of fruits and vegetables. These include potassium, vitamin C, folate, beta carotene, and vitamin E. These are all essentials for protecting the body's cells against oxidative stress and disease.

How to Eat Mediterranean Style

Start with the basics. When you shop, choose whole, fiber-rich foods and make fish and legumes your main sources of protein. Other tips:

• Skip packaged foods and foods high in sugar.
• Choose healthy sources of fat, like the monounsaturated fats in olive oil and avocados.
• Add roasted vegetables to all your lunches and dinners. You'll love all the flavor!
• Add olives and sunflower seeds to your salads.
• Upgrade your snacking to nuts and seeds.
• Enjoy fruit, like a bowl of berries, rather than a junk dessert.

What you eat matters, but how you eat does too. Along with eating the right foods, follow the traditional Mediterranean eating habits, which include eating smaller meals and snacking less. Eat slowly and mindfully and focus on the taste and texture of each bite. Also, buy your food locally whenever possible from smaller farms where you know the growers and can establish a relationship with them.

The Bottom Line

Eating a Mediterranean diet is easy and delicious. It's also healthy for you! So, you have lots of reasons to adopt this style of diet. Have fun exploring the wonderful world of Mediterranean foods.

TIP #53: THREE REASONS WHY YOU SHOULD HAVE A WEEKLY CHEAT MEAL

Snacking on chocolate chip cookies and pizza may not seem like the best way to lose weight, but incorporating a cheat day into your diet can help you slim down. Here are three reasons why.

1. Cheat Days for Leptin Release

Fat cells release a hormone called leptin that tells the hypothalamus in the brain to suppress hunger and speed up metabolism. When you lose fat, you have less tissue to produce leptin, which stimulates appetite. During periods of prolonged dieting, leptin levels also decrease, which slows metabolism and makes it harder to lose weight. By including a weekly cheat day high in carbohydrates, you stimulate a release of insulin, which also increases leptin release.

2. Cheat Days as a Mental Break

Dieting for long periods of time is mentally draining. By breaking up your diet with a weekly cheat day, you may be less likely to quit your diet. Having a cheat day also means you don't need to cut out foods that you love. It also serves as a reward for sticking to your diet and gives you something to look forward to at the end of the week.

3. Cheat Days for Your Social Life

Having a cheat day built into your weekly diet allows you to have more freedom in your social life. For example, if you are going to your friend's wedding on a Saturday night, you can enjoy food that's high in sugar without having to feel guilty. Your cheat day also doesn't have to be on the same day each week. If you have a party coming up on a Friday night but the week before you cheated on Saturday, you can switch your cheat day to fit your social calendar. However, be careful if you decide to move your cheat day to the beginning of the week, or else you may have to go almost two weeks before your next one.

Conclusion

Nutrition timing is an integral part of any diet. By having a cheat day once a week, you can still enjoy your favorite foods and use the extra carbs to keep your metabolism high. If you don't think you can control yourself for an entire day without binge eating, you can also limit yourself to a cheat meal instead.

TIP #54: THREE EASY TIPS FOR MAKING HEALTHY FOOD CHOICES

Are you in the habit of making terrible food choices? This is a great time to make a change. Use this fresh beginning to make healthy food choices for the new year. The following suggestions can help you make a great start.

1) Eat your Veggies.
A diet rich in vegetables not only provides a plethora of vitamins and minerals to nourish your body, but it also helps keep your weight at healthy levels.

Vegetables are necessary to keep the digestive system balanced, because most of them provide a gentle source of fiber to help keep it functioning at its peak. Veggies also provide a large array of essential nutrients for the body, from vitamins A, C and D (which help build healthy skin and bones) all the way to folic acid and potassium (which are great for maintaining healthy heart function). Healthy dining for the new year requires an abundance of vegetables on your dinner plate.

2) Do you have a weakness for sweets?
Put aside the snack cakes and candy bars! Choose to eat healthy by enjoying fruits instead. Some fruits may contain minimal amounts of fat, but the nutritional benefits you will reap far outweigh any fat calories that will be consumed.

Fruits provide natural sugars that will satisfy your sweet tooth, as well as vitamins and minerals that are essential for a healthy body. Make a healthy food choice by replacing sugar-laden, processed sweets with nutrient-packed, beneficial fruits.

3) Choose Healthy Meats.

Some of the top choices in this category include salmon, chicken and lean cuts of pork. Each of these provides your body with low amounts of fat and relatively few calories, while also providing nutrients such as magnesium, potassium, iron, niacin and protein. Proper portion sizes vary, but a good rule of thumb is to compare the serving of meat on your plate to the size of a deck of playing cards or a bar of bath soap. If your meat portion is in this size range, it is most likely an acceptable serving amount.

These are just a few ways you can make healthy food choices for the new year. You can add a few sunflowers seeds to a green salad, snack on almonds between meals and wash down a nutritious breakfast with a glass of pomegranate juice. The options are endless.

Making healthy food choices takes focus. Don't let yourself get derailed. Even dining at fast food restaurants offers no excuse for making poor food choices, because many of them offer salads, fruits and juices.

Remember this is the only body you've got. Keep it healthy! Eat nutritious veggies freely, satisfy your craving for sweets with nutrient-packed fruits and choose healthy, lean meats. There's no better way to start the new year than by choosing to eat healthy.

TIP #55: HONEY VS. SUGAR – WHICH IS BETTER FOR THE BODY?

As the focus for weight loss and healthy living shifts from dietary fats to sugars, more and more people are looking for alternatives to refined white sugar (sucrose). Artificial sweeteners such as aspartame and saccharine once proclaimed as being the calorie- and carb-free answer are falling from favor as various health-related concerns arise. Of the natural sweeteners honey (fructose and glucose) is the only one that can be easily used as is. Others, such as rebaudioside A and xylitol must be extracted from their natural sources and are generally combined with other additives before being sold as sweeteners or added to commercial products. So, how does honey stack up against sugar?

Calories and Carbohydrates

A teaspoon of honey contains 22 calories while an equal amount of table sugar contains only 16. Since honey is considerably sweeter than sugar, due to the fructose, less is used, so the total calories required to achieve the same level of sweetness are approximately the same. As far as carbohydrates are concerned, things even out with one teaspoon of both honey and sugar containing approximately five grams.

Glycemic Index and Load

The glycemic index, which measures how quickly a carbohydrate raises your blood sugar, is significantly lower for honey (55) is than it is for sugar (68). When the glycemic load (which takes into account the total amount of carbohydrates in the food) is taken into account things even out with both honey (9) and sugar (8) coming in on the low end of the scale.

Nutritional Value

Table sugar contains no nutrients whatsoever, while honey contains a variety of vitamins and minerals including B6, thiamin, niacin, riboflavin, iron, magnesium and zinc. Keep in mind, however, that the amount of these nutrients is extremely small. As an example, you would need to ingest approximately 50 cups of honey to get your daily recommended amount of magnesium.

Dental Health

When it comes to cavities, honey wins the battle hands down. Sugar causes tooth decay, and it looks as if honey may actually prevent it. A New Zealand study showed that honey consumption actually reduces plaque build-up. Honey contains enzymes that produce hydrogen peroxide, and it is believed that it is the anti-microbial effect of the hydrogen peroxide that prevents bacteria from sticking to teeth, allowing the plaque a place to settle. The study also found that a certain type of honey (Manuka) reduces plaque even after the hydrogen peroxide is removed from the honey. These results have not yet been replicated with other types of honey.

TIP #56: NUTRITIOUS FOODS
FOR YOUR COLON HEALTH

The colon, also known as the large intestine, plays a vital role in how waste food passes from the body. If the bowel does not work correctly, you can suffer from excess gas and bloating. You could also wind up with colorectal cancer. One of the easiest ways to keep your colon healthy is through nutrition.

Legumes such as dried beans, split peas, and lentils have a lot of fiber. Bean fiber is known to be the best fiber for your colon. Legumes also have phytochemicals, which can protect cells from genetic damage and prevent cancer. Beans also are rich in healthy carbohydrates. Since your body cannot break down these carbs, they will ferment in your colon and churn out anti-cancer compounds. Include lima, navy, kidney, pinto, and even baked beans in your diet regularly.

Flavonols are antioxidants that are known to fight colon cancer. Flavonols can stop cancer cells from forming as well as help keep it from returning. These compounds can prevent cancer growth by extinguishing inflammation. Yellow onions, broccoli, kale, apples, and leeks are among the best sources. Most diets do not include enough of these foods so make a habit of adding more on your plate.

Cruciferous vegetables have compounds such as sulforaphane and indole-3-carbinol. Eating these vegetables can help kill damaged cells and prevent them from turning cancerous. Consuming them raw will provide the most benefit but eating them cooked help. You might have to eat more for the same benefit. Crucifers include broccoli, cauliflower, kale, brussels sprouts, and cabbage.

Whole grain foods are better for your colon than refined grains. Wild and brown rice, quinoa, barley, oatmeal and whole wheat flour fall in this category. These grains have the vitamins, minerals, antioxidants, phytochemicals, and fiber necessary for a healthy colon.

Calcium and vitamin D are thought to give you a lower risk of colon cancer. Just make sure that you do not get too much calcium as that can be bad for you. Try for 1000 to 1300 milligrams per day, depending on your age. To get that amount, you would need to drink three or four cups of milk. Of course, you can always substitute yogurt, cheese, or dark leafy greens such as spinach and kale to get your required calcium intake.

Most colon cancers are not hereditary, but due to lifestyle choices. Eating healthy foods is vital to keeping your colon working as it should. Include the foods mentioned here to help you stay well and avoid cancer or other problems of the colon.

TIP #57: SEVEN FOODS THAT NATURALLY BOOST FERTILITY

Fertility is affected by a large number of internal and external factors, not the least of which is your diet. Even at a healthy body weight, nutrients in the food that you eat can have a significant impact on your ability to conceive. Below are some of the foods that anyone considering a child should add to their diet.

Blueberries:
While many types of fruit contain antioxidants, blueberries are considered one of the strongest sources. Antioxidants fight free radicals, which are destructive molecules that can damage sperm and egg DNA. The vitamin C in blueberries has also been linked to increased sperm count and motility in men.

Lean Meats:
Lean meats contain high levels of iron and high-quality protein, which are especially important during conception and pregnancy. Women with iron deficiencies often have a much more difficult time conceiving, and menstruation can make the issue even worse, since iron stores are depleted due to bleeding.

Salmon:
Salmon and other fatty fish, including sardines and mackerel, are a wonderful source of omega-3 fatty acids, an essential nutrient that the body cannot produce on its own. These fatty acids improve sperm count and motility in men, while reducing the risk of premature birth and postpartum depression in women. Salmon poses a much lower mercury risk than many other fish, making it a much safer choice before and during pregnancy.

Walnuts:
Like salmon, walnuts contain omega-3 fatty acids that contribute to increased fertility in both men and women. Walnuts and other nuts are also a good source of fiber and many other vitamins and minerals, including vitamin E, iron, and calcium.

Whole Milk:
Studies show that whole-fat dairy products, such as whole milk, cheese, and even ice cream can all increase the odds of conception. These foods help regulate hormones, resulting in a much lower risk of infertility related to ovulation. However, research also suggests that low-fat dairy offers far fewer benefits, and skim milk may even do more harm than good, so make a conscious effort to stick to whole-fat dairy products whenever possible.

Lentils:
Lentils contain a host of nutrients that contribute to increased fertility. In addition to being a great source of plant-based protein, lentils are also high in iron. Research indicates that women who get the majority of their daily iron from plant sources have significantly lower rates of infertility. The fiber in lentils ensures that it is digested more slowly, allowing your body to reap the maximum benefit from the vitamins and minerals they contain.

Whole Grains:
Whenever possible, choose whole grain foods while trying to conceive. Processing strips grains of many important nutrients, including fiber. Carbohydrates without fiber are digested much more rapidly, which in turn has a negative effect on insulin and blood sugar levels, creating potential hormone imbalances. Whole grains are digested more slowly, in addition to containing much higher levels of iron, B-vitamins, and helpful antioxidants.

Diet and body weight play an important role in fertility for both men and women, so it's absolutely vital to ensure that you are getting enough of the important nutrients when trying to conceive. By incorporating the above foods into your diet -in addition to following the advice given by your chosen healthcare professional--virtually anyone can improve their odds of getting pregnant.

TIP #58: HOW MANY CALORIES DO I NEED TO EAT?

When we are determined to lose weight, we are tempted to cut down the amount of food we eat dramatically. It would seem logical to think that if we reduce our calories then we will lose weight, and whilst this is true in theory, if we cut our calorie intake too much, we may actually not only prevent weight loss but also create other health problems. Calories are essentially units that measure the amount of energy we eat in our food or we use in our daily activities and when we exercise. To maintain a healthy weight, our calories burned during any 24-hour period must not be less than the amount of calories we ingest in our food during that time. Our bodies can compensate for the occasional meal that is very high in calories, but over the course of a few weeks and months, if we continue to eat more than we exercise, we will gain weight.

Balancing our Daily Caloric Needs with Our Desire to Lose Weight

Traditional diets are being replaced by food plans that limit calorie intake to the amount that provides only adequate calories for daily activities. When the body receives fewer calories than it can use as energy, it will begin to burn stored fat to get the energy that it needs. Stored fat is the energy source that the body uses when our food intake does not supply enough calories to provide us with the energy our body needs to function. By limiting intake to a minimum recommended daily calorie intake and increasing the amount of calories burned through exercise, we will lose weight.

Our required caloric intake is dependent upon gender, age, activity level, and other factors. Most good plans will include a checklist to ensure you are eating an appropriate amount of food for your personal requirements. If you have a chronic disease, such as type 2 diabetes or a digestive disorder, you should always check with your doctor first.

Averages for Men and Women

Assuming you are young, fit, and healthy, the suggested calorie intake for a woman who has an average lifestyle is between 1700 to 2000 calories each day. If a woman is pregnant or breastfeeding, calorie requirements rise to around 2300 calories per day. A man who is moderately active will need approximately 2300 to 2500 calories each day. But a very active man may require 3000 or more a day, as a minimum, to stay strong and healthy.

Eating for Weight Loss

Individuals who want to lose weight effectively should reduce the amount of calories they consume by around 500 calories per day, and anyone who wants to lose weight must look at what foods they are consuming to get the necessary calories they need to function each day. Swapping simple carbohydrates, such as potatoes, rice, and white bread, for sweet potatoes, brown rice, and whole grain bread, will help you reduce the calories you ingest by keeping you feeling fuller for longer periods throughout the day. These foods also reduce the swings in blood sugar levels that cause much of the food-related damage to the body over an extended period of time.

There are a number of diet plans that follow these simple guidelines and, in the long run, they almost all work better than the quick faddy diets that unfortunately are so popular right now. Following these recommended daily calorie guides will assist you not only in losing weight but also in maintaining your general health and preventing sneaky weight gain that can develop gradually over many years.

TIP #59: THE IMPORTANCE
OF EATING BREAKFAST

Eating a healthy breakfast is one of the most important things you can do for your body every single day. In addition to providing you with energy, there are actually many health benefits to eating a healthy breakfast to start your day. A 2005 study synthesizing 47 studies reports that people who skip breakfast are more likely to start smoking or drinking, are less likely to exercise, and are more likely to express concerns about dieting.

Even more incredible is the fact that breakfast eaters are 30% less likely to be overweight or obese. This means that people who eat breakfast tend to eat more but weigh less. People who eat breakfast jump-start their bodies into earlier metabolism than those who wait until much later to eat their first meal.

The first meal of the day also helps people improve their concentration throughout the day and perform better in school or on the job. Breakfast also provides us with more strength and endurance as we engage in physical activity as the day continues. Fatigue is less likely to set in, especially during the early afternoon hours.

Including lean protein in your breakfast is one of the best ways to maintain a healthy diet routine. Although eggs are not necessarily contributors of lower weight, they are the best source of high-quality protein out there. Eating two eggs at breakfast is much healthier than a bagel, with or without cream cheese.

According to an article in the Journal of the American College of Nutrition, "When people eat eggs at breakfast, they felt more satisfied and consumed fewer calories throughout the day." A slice of Canadian bacon at breakfast time will also do the trick and lead people to feel less hungry during the rest of the morning.

Breakfast cereals have also been found to potentially play a major role in maintaining a healthy weight. Cereals of the whole-grain types are the best. People who eat cereals regularly for breakfast were found to weigh less than those who skipped breakfast all together.

Many people skip breakfast because they claim they do not have any time to eat. Some quick and healthy ideas for breakfast include:
- a smoothie made with low-fat yogurt and fruit
- a hard-boiled egg and a banana or other fruit
- whole-grained cereal with low-fat milk and fresh fruit
- a Canadian bacon omelet and whole-wheat toast

Eating a healthy breakfast helps prevent your body from hitting rock bottom and getting too hungry. By noon, when your brain and body are running on empty and have no glucose left, they are no longer able to function properly and at their potentials. Your brain loses focus and has a hard time concentrating. Your body goes into starvation mode and starts to store as much as it can, in the form of fat, thinking it will not be getting anything good anytime soon. This is why people who skip meals tend to gain weight rather than lose it.

Breakfast is a great time to consume the important nutrients your body needs to stay healthy. Essential vitamins and minerals, which help build bone strength and a healthy immune system, are plentiful in breakfast foods. Most importantly, breakfast is the best time to replenish blood glucose to levels needed for proper brain and body function.

It is, in fact, true when people say, "Breakfast is the most important meal of the day." Not only is it the meal that breaks the fast between dinner the night before and the meal you will eat after you have started your day, it is the one that sets the tone for the rest of the day. Breakfast gives you the energy boost needed to have a productive, focused day at work or at play.

TIP #60: QUICK AND HEALTHY BREAKFASTS

You know that breakfast is important. Scientific studies suggest that eating a healthy breakfast may improve your performance at work and school and reduce your chances of obesity and certain chronic diseases. A 2013 study from the Harvard School of Public Health, for example, suggests skipping breakfast may increase your risk of heart disease. Just knowing the importance of a healthy breakfast isn't enough. For most people, the issue on weekdays is finding time to make and eat breakfast after hitting the snooze button on your alarm, spilling coffee on your clothes, getting distracted by cat pictures when doing a quick check of e-mail, or hunting for misplaced car keys. Even if you don't have time for a cooked breakfast, you don't need to eat an artery-clogging breakfast pastry or skip breakfast entirely. Below are several quick, healthy, no-fuss, no-mess breakfast options you can eat on the run.

Breakfast Nutrition

Breakfast traditions vary tremendously. The French have their croissants, the Japanese, rice and miso soup, the Chinese, dumplings or noodle soup, and the British, a cooked breakfast including sausages, bacon, mushrooms, cooked tomatoes, and black pudding. You can eat almost any food you enjoy for breakfast as long as it contains a balance of lean proteins and good carbohydrates such as whole grains or fresh fruits or vegetables. Most adults should aim to consume 350 to 500 calories or approximately 25 to 35 percent of their total daily calories at breakfast, including at least 15 to 20 grams of protein. Avoid refined carbohydrates and sugars, as they give a quick energy surge followed by a sharp energy drop just when you need to be alert and attentive at work or school.

Sandwiches
The original convenience food, the sandwich, was named after an eighteenth-century nobleman, John Montagu, the fourth Earl of Sandwich, an avid gambler who would have his servant bring him meat layered between two slices of bread so he could eat dinner without interrupting his card game. Make your own healthy breakfast sandwiches at home with whole grain or multi-grain bread or pita, filled with proteins such as hummus, nut butters, cheese, meat, or eggs. If you grab breakfast sandwiches at a local drive-through, check nutritional information online to find healthy choices.

Eggs
With 80 calories and 6 grams of protein, eggs are breakfast standards in North America and Britain. For an instant healthy breakfast, prepare hard-boiled eggs at night and just peel and eat two for breakfast along with a piece of fresh fruit. Hard-boiled eggs will last for up to a week in your refrigerator, so you can make a batch on Sunday night and have an instant breakfast ready for busy weekdays.

Smoothies and Shakes
Smoothies and shakes make a perfect no-mess, on-the-go breakfast. Before you go to bed, you can make a traditional smoothie in the blender with fruit, ice cubes, and protein powder and then store it in the refrigerator overnight. Another option is tossing ice cubes, protein powder, soy or skim milk, and perhaps fruit juice into a tumbler or water bottle and shaking for an instant breakfast. Combine your morning caffeine with your breakfast protein in a delicious mocha shake by adding a cup of cold coffee, ice-cubes, two scoops of chocolate- or carob-flavored protein powder, and skim or soy milk to a tumbler and shaking vigorously. For extra fiber and omega-3s, add ground flax seeds to your shake or smoothie.

Fruit, Nuts, and Cheese

Two ounces of cheese will supply 10 grams of protein. Try hard cheeses on apple or pear slices for a refreshing start to your day. If you're having the sort of morning where even slicing fruit and cheese will make you late, keep around individual packets of string cheese and small sandwich bags filled with grapes or mini-carrots for a grab-and-go meal. Although nuts can be high in calories, in limited quantities they are a healthy quick breakfast or snack, with a half cup of raw almonds containing 10 grams of protein and close to your complete daily requirement of vitamin E and biotin.

Protein Bars

The ultimate in convenience food, protein bars can be stashed in your briefcase or glove compartment for a no-mess instant breakfast. Read nutrition information carefully, as many are filled with refined sugar and fat, and are no healthier than a piece of candy. The other problem is that because most meal bars are small and have only minimal amounts of fiber, they may leave you feeling hungry, leaving you susceptible to doughnuts or other unhealthy break room treats. While not a perfect choice, a small stash of protein bars will help you get through the most hectic of mornings.

BOOKS BY THIS AUTHOR

50 Simple Ways To Eat Better

50 Powerful Exercise Benefits And Tips

130 Reasons Why You Struggle To Lose Weight And How To Fix Them

65 Simple Tips For A Healthy Lifestyle